ESCAPING EMOTIONAL ABUSE

Healing from the Shame You Don't Deserve

BEVERLY ENGEL, LMFT

CITADEL PRESS
Kensington Publishing Corp.
www.kensingtonbooks.com

CITADEL PRESS BOOKS are published by

Kensington Publishing Corp.
119 West 40th Street
New York, NY 10018

All Kensington titles, imprints, and distributed lines are available at special quantity discounts for bulk purchases for sales promotions, premiums, fund-raising, educational, or institutional use. Special book excerpts or customized printings can also be created to fit specific needs. For details, write or phone the office of the Kensington sales manager: Kensington Publishing Corp., 119 West 40th Street, New York, NY 10018, attn: Sales Department; phone 1-800-221-2647.

CITADEL PRESS and the Citadel logo are Reg. U.S. Pat. & TM Off.

ISBN-13: 978-0-8065-4050-4
ISBN-10: 0-8065-4050-8

First Citadel printing: January 2021

10 9 8 7 6 5 4 3 2 1

Printed in the United States of America

Electronic edition:

ISBN-13: 978-0-8065-4051-1 (e-book)
ISBN-10: 0-8065-4051-6 (e-book)

Praise for

Escaping Emotional Abuse

"A warm, compassionate, and incredibly insightful guide through the recovery journey. Engel's words are a powerful antidote to the seemingly unshakeable shame that comes from emotional abuse. There is hope, healing, and wisdom to be found on every page."

—Jackson MacKenzie, author of *Psychopath Free*

"An extremely informative and comprehensive guide to understanding and overcoming emotional abuse. Beverly Engel gives you all the information you need to stop blaming yourself and get back control of your life."

—Lundy Bancroft, author of *Why Does He Do That?*

"I highly recommend this book for anyone—female or male—who suspects they are being emotionally abused. I especially appreciate the information on how emotional abuse can be shaming, which is dangerous to a person's self-esteem and sense of self."

—Randi Kreger, co-author of *Stop Walking on Eggshells* and author of *The Essential Guide to Borderline Personality Disorder*

"Written with love and expertise, *Escaping Emotional Abuse* is a comprehensive and compassionate guidebook for victims of abuse. It provides a road map to healing from the entanglement of shame and abuse that imprisons victims and binds them to perpetrators."

—Darlene Lancer, LMFT, author of *Conquering Shame and Codependency*

I dedicate this book to all my past and present clients.
Your courage and determination inspire me every day.

You were born with potential. You were born with good-ness and trust. You were born with ideals and dreams. You were born with greatness. You were born with wings. You are not meant for crawling, so don't. You have wings. Learn to use them and fly.

—RUMI

Contents

Escaping Emotional Abuse

Introduction

BELIEVE THIS IS one of the most important books I've written. Although I've been working with victims of emotional abuse for over thirty-five years and have written four books on the subject, I found that there was still more that I needed to offer my readers.

Emotional abuse is one of the most difficult types of abuse to identify because it is so hidden, insidious, and confusing. The damage caused by emotional abuse, while significant, can occur so slowly that the victim hardly notices it at first. Like the abuse itself, the damage can be so subtle that it is easy for victims to minimize it, deny it, or believe they are imagining it. So helping people recognize that they are being emotionally abused is important. But it is not the entire answer to the problem.

Time after time, I have observed that even when people realize they are being emotionally abused, they aren't necessarily prepared to end the relationship. This is because most victims of emotional abuse suffer from horrible, debilitating shame—shame that robs them of their motivation to take action, shame that prevents them from believing they deserve anything better.

As important as it is to discover that you are being emotionally abused and how it is damaging you, it is equally important to be able to work past your shame. Unless you recognize your shame and begin to heal it, your hands will feel tied in terms of being able to escape your relationship. Shame will cause you to curl up and make yourself feel smaller at a time when you need to stand up

3

and feel empowered. It will cause you to blame yourself for your partner's actions and to feel bad about how you have reacted to the abuse at times.

I realized that I needed to send a strong message that lets victims of emotional abuse know that it is understandable that it can be extremely difficult to end their abusive relationship, even when they know they need to do so. I needed to help them stop blaming themselves for the abuse, and even more important, I needed to help them realize that they deserved to be treated with consideration and respect.

Until recently, shame was one of the least understood emotions. People don't connect with their shame in the way they can connect with their anger or their sadness or their fear. But for those who are being emotionally abused, shame is the most important emotion to identify and connect with. This is because shame is the reason most people stay in an abusive relationship.

Whatever you choose to do—to stay in your relationship or end it—in order to gain the courage, strength, and determination to either confront an abuser and/or end an emotionally abusive relationship, you need to rid yourself of your shame.

Shame is by far the most destructive aspect of emotional abuse, and it can be the most difficult to heal. It causes victims to stay in an abusive relationship because it makes them feel so bad about themselves that they come to believe that no one else would ever want them. When you are consistently shamed, you come to feel you are worthless and unlovable, that you are damaged beyond repair. Add this to the shame victims feel because they are unable to stand up to the abuser or walk away from the relationship and you can see how emotional abuse creates a *prison of shame*. Just as surely as someone who is locked up behind bars has no freedom and very little choice, victims of emotional abuse also feel trapped and powerless.

Escaping the prison of shame that confines you and continues to wear you down is not an easy task. You will need to learn that the abuse is not your fault—a monumental task in itself. Then you need to begin to believe that you deserve to be treated with more respect and consideration—another monumental task. Next, you need to be able to shore up your confidence in order to begin to stand up for yourself, name the abuse, and set boundaries. Finally, you may need to shore up even more confidence in order to walk away from the abuser, often someone you still love. In this book, I will guide you step-by-step through a program that will help you complete all these difficult tasks—a program that will help you to heal your shame, free yourself from the clutches of an abusive partner, and become more empowered.

And there are still two more important things this book will offer you: support and encouragement.

Emotional abuse is a very isolating experience. Your partner may have discouraged you from seeing your family and friends, or you may have so much shame about being abused that you have distanced yourself from them on your own. You may have opened up to someone only to discover that he or she was critical of you for not leaving, or the reverse, critical of you for considering leaving. Either way, you probably didn't get the support you needed. You may feel that no one you know will be able to understand your situation. But I *do* understand. I spent my childhood being emotionally abused. I didn't understand this, of course. All I knew was that I felt constantly confused because I could never please my mother no matter how hard I tried. I was convinced that there was something terribly wrong with me. And I had absolutely no one to talk to. I was utterly alone.

I want you to know that you are not alone. And I want you to know that no matter what you decide to do, I will support you.

When you think of what is involved in escaping your prison of shame, it can seem to be a daunting task. But I will walk alongside you on your journey—from shame and fear to self-compassion and inner strength. My program will make this seemingly impossible journey a reality.

The comprehensive program I offer you has been carefully designed to take you from learning about emotional abuse and its effects to finding out how you can extricate yourself from your partner's lies, manipulation, and criticism. It's a process that will help you decide whether to stay in the relationship or end it, and if you do leave, it will help you to avoid going back. Most important, this program will help you heal the shame of abuse.

My highly effective Shame Reduction Program was developed to help my clients who suffered from what I call "debilitating shame." It features five major avenues for reducing or eliminating the shame of emotional abuse:

1. **Emotional abuse deprogramming:** Many victims of emotional abuse have been brainwashed and need to be deprogrammed. I provide information and strategies to accomplish this much-needed process.

2. **Anger expression:** Whereas shame depletes our energy, anger energizes and empowers. Anger can help you begin to feel less helpless and hopeless and begin to feel more empowered. It can help you become less fearful of your abuser and may even help you to imagine standing up to your abuser. And perhaps most important, it will help you to give your shame back to your abuser. I will offer strategies to help you overcome any fear you have about getting angry and techniques to use to release your anger in healthy and safe ways.

3. **Self-compassion:** As it is with most poisons, the toxicity of shame needs to be neutralized by another substance if we are truly going to save the patient. Compassion is the only thing that can neutralize shame. Self-compassion will teach you how to develop *an internal compassionate relationship with yourself* in order to counter the shame you have experienced due to emotional abuse. You will learn specific compassionate attitudes and skills that can re-

verse your tendency to blame yourself for the abuse and help you begin to understand that you did nothing to deserve the abuse. In addition, it will help you to understand why you have stayed in the relationship and to forgive yourself for the negative behaviors you may have exhibited in response to your abuse experiences—everything from alcohol and drug abuse to being reckless with yourself and your body. Finally, self-compassion will help you to give yourself the nurturance, understanding, and validation you so desperately need in order to feel worthy of care, respect, and acceptance. For all these reasons, self-compassion will be an important focus of the book and a primary strategy for healing shame.

4. **Self-forgiveness:** Self-forgiveness is a powerful way to reduce or even eliminate shame. In this section, I will guide you step-by-step through the process of completing the major tasks related to self-forgiveness. First and foremost, those who have been shamed or abused need to forgive themselves for the abuse itself. Second, they need to forgive themselves for remaining in the relationship and for harm they caused their children and others. And finally, they need to forgive themselves for the harm they have caused themselves.

5. **Self-kindness:** Unfortunately, shame has probably kept many readers from feeling kind toward themselves in much the same way that it may have been difficult to accept kindness from others. You may not believe you deserve to be treated with the same patience, tenderness, and comfort that you might naturally feel for a loved one. Hopefully, the tools in this book will change that perception. You might not even know how to treat yourself with loving kindness, but if you can come to believe you deserve it, then this book will help you learn how to practice it.

In addition to helping you reduce your shame, I will address your fears and insecurities about what to do next. Should you end the relationship? After all, you made a commitment to this person. Should you confront your partner and hope he or she will be able to recognize his or her abusive behavior and work toward changing it? Is it okay to give up on a person when he or she had such a horrible childhood? And there are other questions as well: Can I make it on my own? Is it right to take my children away from their other parent? These are difficult questions for anyone to consider, but they are questions that need answers.

He or She?

As you read the book, you will notice that some case examples identify the victim as being female while others are male. You will also notice that while most examples are of heterosexual couples, there will also be a few examples of homosexual couples. I include these examples because I want everyone—no matter what his or her sex, sexual orientation, or gender identity—to know that emotional abuse occurs in all kinds of relationships.

It doesn't matter if you are rich or poor, college educated, working outside the home, or a fulltime caregiver and parent, emotional abuse can happen to you. A major goal of this book is to take the shame out of emotional abuse, including the shame surrounding not being able to admit that you are a victim of this kind of mistreatment.

Why I Use the Word *Victim* Instead of *Survivor*

As you may have already noticed, I use the word *victim* when describing someone who is being emotionally abused. I do this deliberately because I want you to recognize that you are, in fact, being victimized by your partner.

It can be very difficult to admit that you are a victim of emotional abuse—or a victim of anything, for that matter. Any time someone is victimized, he or she feels helpless, and the feeling of helplessness causes us to feel humiliated. Acknowledging that you are being victimized can make you feel weak and less than other people. Many think of the word *victim* as a dirty word, synonymous with weakness or being a "loser," but the actual definition of *victim* is "a person harmed, injured, or killed as a result of a crime, accident, or other event or action." In our victim-hating and victim-blaming culture, the term *victim* has become more of an insult than an accurate identifier that indicates a person has endured a trauma at the hands of another person (or persons). We have bastardized the word to the point that it is used to diminish, discredit, and disparage anyone who has endured the worst of humanity.

I use the word *victim* deliberately because I don't want to minimize the abuse that you are experiencing. At this point, you are, in fact, a victim and all that implies. You are a victim of your partner's emotional abuse, and you are a victim to the debilitating shame that comes with the experience of being abused. In admitting that you are a victim of emotional abuse, you are actually taking the first step toward healing because you can't heal what you don't acknowledge.

It has become politically correct to use the word *survivor* instead of *victim* when describing someone who was abused and has survived the experience. The argument is that this term is more empowering than the word *victim*, and I completely agree. But as far as I am concerned, until you are able to either confront your abuser or end the relationship, you are still a victim.

According to Merriam-Webster, there are two main definitions of survivor: (1) "to remain alive or in existence" and (2) "to continue to function or prosper." The truth is, *survivor* doesn't really describe how most people who are being emotionally abused would describe their ongoing experience with their partner. Sure, they are still alive, and they are still functioning, but I would hardly say that they are "prospering" or functioning at their optimum.

I believe that the word *survivor* can paint a misleading picture of victimhood and healing. It encourages victims to "get over it" instead of addressing and having compassion for their suffering, an important step in healing. Once you are able to heal your shame enough to stand up to your abuser or to end the relationship, you will be on the path to becoming a survivor.

Over the years, I have received feedback from many clients who are actually offended when someone calls them a survivor, especially when they are just beginning to heal from the abuse. They told me that they want to be the one to decide what they call themselves and that the word *survivor* doesn't fit for them until they have experienced some substantial recovery. Another objection to being called a survivor by others is that they feel that their victimization is being glossed over—that the word *survivor* makes other people more comfortable than admitting that the person was victimized.

For the most part, I am going to use the word *victim* to describe those adults who are being emotionally abused. It's not that I don't want you to feel empowered. And it's not that I don't give you credit for surviving horrific abuse, but I want you to acknowledge to yourself that you are indeed being victimized by your partner.

If you have a strong reaction to the word *victim*, I ask you to question why this is. Is it possible that you are still struggling with the fact that you are, in fact, being victimized? Is it because deep down inside you are still blaming yourself? Is it that you hate the idea of being victimized because you think that victims are weak, that they are losers?

If the answer to any of these questions is yes, my hope is that this book will help you to rethink these self-defeating ideas. My hope is that you will come to see that it is not a weakness to be a victim; it is only a sign that you are human. All of us are victimized sometime in our lives, most people many times. We can't prevent ourselves from being victimized, but we can admit it to ourselves, understand that we don't deserve it, have compassion for our suffering, and use the strategies we need to exorcise ourselves from an abusive situation. This book will help you to do all these things.

PART I

THE CONNECTION BETWEEN SHAME AND EMOTIONAL ABUSE

CHAPTER 1

Emotional Abuse and Shame— A Perfect Marriage

Her body was a prison, her mind was a prison. Her mem-
ories were a prison. The people she loved. She couldn't
get away from the hurt of them....Tonight even the sky
felt like a prison.

—ANN BRASHARES, *Sisterhood Everlasting*

IF YOU ARE IN AN emotionally abusive relationship, you may feel as if you are in prison. You aren't free to conduct your life the way you choose because you always have to answer to someone. You are always afraid of "doing something wrong" and being chastised for it. And you always have to explain yourself and your motives.

Your partner may have a need to control all aspects of your life: what you spend money on, how much you spend, how you dress, whom you associate with. He or she may be overly possessive and jealous, accusing you of flirting or, worse, accusing you of having affairs. You may feel like you can't do anything without risking being criticized or being falsely accused of something.

Because of all this, you feel trapped, unable to escape, unable to even imagine how to do so. You may feel like you can't tolerate living with your partner one more day, and yet you may be afraid that you will not be able to live without him or her. You may feel like anything has to be better than this, but you also are afraid it actually could be worse if you try to make it without your partner.

Emotional abuse can create a prison for its victims because even when you know you are being mistreated, you may not have the ability to end the relationship. You may be so worn down from years of abuse that you've lost your self-confidence, your courage, even your will to live.

The purpose of putting someone in prison is to *confine* them, *punish* them, and have *control* of them. Emotional abusers do all these things to their partner, essentially making their partner their prisoner. But it is important to note that people are put in prison because they have "done something wrong." *The truth is, you have done nothing wrong and don't deserve to be punished.* Helping you realize this will be a major goal of this book.

Emotional abuse creates tremendous shame in its victims. If people are emotionally abused long enough and intensely enough, they will come to believe they don't deserve to be respected and loved. They will come to believe they deserve to be treated with disrespect, impatience, contempt, and even cruelty. They will feel humiliated so often that they will come to believe they don't deserve to ask for anything or expect anything from their partner.

PERHAPS YOU RECOGNIZE yourself in this description. You may be very aware that you are in an emotionally abusive relationship, and you may feel tremendous shame because you aren't able to leave your partner. You may suffer every day from the things he or she says and does, and you may be keenly aware that the abuse causes you to feel a great deal of shame.

Or perhaps you only *suspect* that you are being emotionally abused. Or you're not aware of how much shame you are experiencing due to the effects of emotional abuse. In fact, you may feel a great deal of confusion about whether you are being mistreated by your partner, and you may blame yourself for the problems in your relationship.

Whatever your situation, if you are reading this book it is likely that you are confused. So, in addition to being imprisoned by shame, you also may feel imprisoned by confusion. You may be confused as to what emotionally abusive behavior actually is, or you may be confused as to whether you deserve the treatment you are receiving from your partner. You may go back and forth, feeling certain that you are being mistreated one day and questioning whether it is true the next. You may vacillate between blaming yourself completely for the problems in your relationship and suspecting that your partner has emotional problems that cause him to behave as he does.

You may have come to doubt yourself on a very deep level, constantly asking yourself questions such as "Am I making too much out of things?" "Am I overreacting?" or "Am I imagining things?"

You may also be confused as to whether you should end your relationship or keep trying to change it. Or you may know that you should end it but are afraid you will regret your decision.

It is actually very common for those who are being emotionally abused to be confused, and there are many reasons for this. A major symptom of emotional abuse is that you feel *off-balance*, *uncertain*, and *disoriented* a great deal of the time. Often, this is actually a goal of some abusers; they know that if they can keep you confused, they can have more control of you.

Your partner may constantly tell you that there are a multitude of things wrong with you, and you may tend to believe him. Maybe you've heard of emotional abuse and even read about it, and you recognize that some of the ways your partner treats you seem to be emotionally abusive. Yet even so, you may still blame yourself for *causing* him to treat you in these negative ways. That's what your partner tells you. He says he wouldn't lose his temper so much if you'd just do what he asks. He says you hurt him so much that he lashes out at you. He says all he wants is for you to show him you love him by doing the things he asks.

Another one of the goals of this book is to end your confusion. I want you to come to a place where you know for certain whether or not you are being emotionally abused and, if so, where you are able to recognize the damage this emotional abuse is causing you. One of the most significant ways of determining whether you are being emotionally abused is to begin to notice your mental and emotional state. Below is a list of the most common effects of emotional abuse. As you read the list, make note of which of these effects or symptoms apply to you. If you choose to, put a check mark next to the symptoms that describe your present state.

☐ Constant or overwhelming confusion
☐ Feeling "off-balance" or disoriented a great deal of the time
☐ Depression (lack of energy, a feeling of impending doom, unable to find joy or pleasure in life, frequently weepy)
☐ Feelings of hopelessness and despair
☐ Feelings of helplessness
☐ Feeling worthless and/or unlovable
☐ Difficulty concentrating
☐ Difficulty making decisions
☐ Feelings of uncertainty and unpredictability
☐ Feeling out of control
☐ Increased self-criticism
☐ Lowered self-esteem and dwindling self-confidence
☐ Overwhelming guilt
☐ Debilitating shame
☐ Self-destructive behavior (consciously or unconsciously trying to hurt or punish yourself)
☐ Increased feelings of insecurity and fear
☐ Crippling self-doubt
☐ Intense anxiety
☐ Constant fear, hypervigilance
☐ Fear of failure

☐ Chronic state of stress
☐ Lack of sexual interest or feeling
☐ Disconnection from emotions
☐ Disconnection from body (dissociation)
☐ Numbness
☐ Obsessive thoughts
☐ Isolating from others
☐ Signs of trauma (panic attacks, nightmares, flashbacks, post-traumatic stress disorder)
☐ Health problems (especially those resulting from toxic and chronic stress, such as high blood pressure, racing heartbeat, muscle tension and pain). Some researchers theorize that emotional abuse may contribute to the development of conditions such as chronic fatigue syndrome and fibromyalgia.

While some of these symptoms can also be common in other conditions and situations, it is the overall combination of symptoms that is important. If you found that you suffer from many of the above symptoms, that can be a strong indication that you are, in fact, being emotionally abused. If you are already certain that you are being abused, recognizing these effects can be an important reminder of the price you are paying by staying in the relationship.

Many of the above effects of emotional abuse are also symptoms of *depression* (loss of energy or increased fatigue; feelings of worthlessness, helplessness, and hopelessness; inappropriate guilt; and difficulty thinking, concentrating, or making decisions). So it is important to note that many of the behaviors you are most critical of, and are likely criticized by your partner for, are actually the *result of emotional abuse*! In other words, it makes perfect sense that you would behave in these ways given the treatment you are receiving!

Although it can be overwhelming to recognize just how many of these symptoms you are suffering from, it can also be life-changing. You may or may not have noticed these symptoms, but even if you did, you probably didn't put two and two together; you didn't realize these symptoms could be related to the way your partner is treating you. This realization may be just the impetus you need to determine that you need to do something about your situation.

The Connection Between Shame and Emotional Abuse

This brings us to the primary focus of this book: the connection between shame and emotional abuse. *Shame is, by far, the most damaging effect of emotional abuse.* Shame damages a victim's self-esteem to the point that she or he loses self-confidence and the ability to see the truth about a situation. Worse yet, shame can also cause a person to believe she or he deserves to be mistreated.

Shame is one of the most destructive weapons used by abusers and can be the most effective. Emotional abusers use shame as a way of gaining control of the victim and the relationship. This shaming slowly whittles away at the victim's self-esteem and self-confidence and makes her question her perceptions and, eventually, her very sanity. Weakened, worn down, and confused, the victim loses her ability to fight back. Even when victims become aware that they are being emotionally abused, many have come to believe that no one else would ever want them or that they can't make it on their own without the abuser. This, in turn, adds to their shame. They chastise themselves with statements like "How can I be so weak that I stay with someone who abuses me like this?" and "What is wrong with me?" Many hide the fact that they are being abused from their family and friends due to shame, and keeping this secret creates even more shame. Soon you have an environment of shame—a prison of shame.

Some forms of emotional abuse are more shaming than others. This includes:

- **Being humiliated**, especially in front of others. "How could you have forgotten to pick up the cake? What kind of mother are you?"
- **Being dismissed.** "That's a ridiculous idea."
- **Being diminished.** "So you won an essay contest; there were only ten other contestants."
- **Being belittled.** "You think you are so smart, don't you? Don't you know that most people can do what you do with their hands tied behind their back?"
- **Being degraded or demeaned.** "You look like a slut in that dress."
- **Being ridiculed.** "Oh, poor baby, you don't feel good. Do you need a bottle?"
- **Exposing your mistakes**, constantly throwing them in your face. "Remember, you are the one who got us in this mess in the first place."
- **Comparing you to others** in a negative way. "I wish you had the kind of well-paying job that your sister has. I wouldn't have to work so hard."
- **Constantly making you wrong.** "Why can't you ever do anything right? I told you this wasn't a good time to paint that room."
- **Being impossible to please.** "When will you ever learn how to cook? This is crap."
- **Making insulting comments.** "Your hair looks ridiculous."
- **Gaslighting.** "I can't believe how much you were flirting with Tom last night at the party. You should be ashamed of yourself." (When you weren't flirting at all.)
- **Emotional blackmail.** "If you aren't willing to do it, I'll find someone who will." (Referring to a sexual practice.)

Verbal abuse is the most common form of emotional abuse and can be the most shame inducing. It is frequently unrecognized because it is often subtle and insidious. It can come under the guise of "advice" or "guidance," and it may be said in a loving voice, quiet voice or be indirect, such as being concealed as a joke. In addition to the forms of verbal abuse listed above, here is a partial list of behaviors that are considered verbally abusive:

- Calling you names
- Insulting you
- Mocking you or making fun of you
- Putting you down
- Trivializing your needs and desires (invalidation)
- Rejecting your opinions
- Accusing you of doing things you haven't done
- Being overly sarcastic with you
- Disparaging your ideas
- Discounting your opinions and ideas
- Undermining and interrupting you
- Denying doing something he or she obviously did
- Threatening you
- Intimidating you

All of these forms of verbal abuse except for the last three are done for the sole purpose of shaming the victim. Abusers usually utilize the last three items to defend themselves or to silence you.

Refusal to be pleased is another particularly shaming form of emotional abuse. Case in point, my client Brandy:

> My husband always complained about my weight. He'd say things to me like, "Are you eating again?" and "You're getting as fat as your sisters." He told me he was no longer attracted to me sexually and that he was ashamed to be seen with me. I wanted my husband to find me attractive, and I felt horrible about myself that he wasn't. I became extremely self-conscious and stopped going places because I was certain other

people were looking at me critically. I finally felt so ashamed of myself that I went on a diet and started walking every day. I lost a lot of weight, and I started feeling better about myself than I had since we had gotten married. But instead of being happy about my weight loss, he started complaining about how men were flirting with me. I felt so defeated. I'd wanted to please him so much, and yet he still found something wrong with me.

Then he started accusing me of flirting with other men. I didn't believe I was, but he was so convincing I began to wonder whether it was true. After all, I did like it when other men found me attractive. Then he accused me of having an affair. No matter how much I denied it, he kept on. He started checking up on me, calling me all day at work, getting angry when I was only a few minutes late from work. I hated it that losing the weight had made him feel so insecure, so I stopped walking every day and started gaining the weight back. But this didn't stop him from accusing me of having an affair. And he even started complaining about my weight again. When that happened, I began to realize I was never going to please him no matter what I did. He was always going to find something wrong with me. I think he gets off on shaming me—making me feel bad about myself.

Emotional abuse and shame go hand in hand—a perfect marriage, so to speak. Shame is a primary factor in emotional abuse since shame is the cause of emotionally abusive behavior, the primary damage caused by emotional abuse, and the primary tool used by abusers. *Coming to identify how shame is affecting you and understanding how shame works to diminish you will be taking the first step toward escaping from your prison.*

Physical Abuse Versus Emotional Abuse

While physical abuse is an attack on the body, emotional abuse is an assault on the psyche and on the soul. The damage done by emotional abuse is deeper and more life-changing than physical abuse and causes the victim to question the truth about herself— to doubt her worthiness as a person, her ability to satisfy a partner, even her ability to love someone else.

In many ways, emotional abuse is more harmful than physical abuse. The main reason for this is that physical abuse is cyclical. There is a violent outburst that is followed by a honeymoon period of remorse, attention, affection, and generosity. Emotional abuse, on the other hand, happens every day. The effects are more harmful because they are so frequent and because there is no downtime to emotionally heal.

Another reason why emotional abuse is more harmful than physical abuse is that there is a greater likelihood that victims will blame themselves. If someone hits you, it's easier to see that he or she is the problem, but if the abuse is subtle—such as saying or implying that you are ugly, a bad parent, stupid, or incompetent, or that no one else could love you—you are more likely to think it's *your* problem. *One of this book's most powerful messages is that you need to begin to question and eventually reject the negative, shaming messages that are not only untrue but are, in fact, emotionally abusive.*

Finally, it is important to know that victims of emotional abuse often suffer from more severe aftereffects than those who experience physical abuse. They are more likely to experience higher rates of anxiety and depression and to have higher rates of PTSD, and they tend to have a more difficult time trusting others in the future, as well as being more likely to have recurring unhealthy relationships. (It is important to note that physical abuse and emotional abuse can go hand in hand, depending on the abuser and the circumstances.)

Escaping the Prison of Self-Criticism and Self-Doubt

Even though you may realize you are being emotionally abused, you may still feel trapped in your relationship, unable to change it or end it. You may have tried everything: talking to your partner about the way he treats you, trying to ignore his words and behavior, even threatening to leave if he doesn't change. You may realize you need to leave your partner and yet find that you are unable to do so, and because of this, you may believe that you are weak or stupid or that something is terribly wrong with you. You may have even left in the past but returned when you found yourself missing him, doubting yourself, or having a difficult time making it on your own. You may not only feel imprisoned in your relationship but also imprisoned by what you consider to be a lack of courage.

Another one of my goals in this book is to not only help you escape the prison of emotional abuse and shame but also your prison of *self-criticism* and *self-doubt*. In these pages, you will not only become clearer about what emotional abuse is but also learn how it slowly eats away at your self-esteem and self-confidence to the point that you doubt yourself, your perceptions, your beliefs, even your sanity. You will learn how to extricate yourself from a partner who treats you badly even though you still love him. And most important, you will learn that you deserve a much better life—a life free of being told how unattractive, lazy, selfish, incompetent, and stupid you are. A life in which you are free to make your own choices and decisions and know they are the right ones for you. A life in which you are free to figure out what you want and what you need instead of always considering your partner's needs first. A life in which you can feel good about yourself, not because you have pleased your partner but because you have pleased yourself.

It is my hope that in these pages you will begin to believe in yourself and in your right to be happy. You will come to stop believing in the complaints and insults told to you by your abusive partner and instead begin to believe in the truth about yourself. You are not stupid, you are not selfish, you are not incompetent or lazy. Those are lies that have been told to you by someone who wants and needs to keep you down and keep you imprisoned in the relationship. In this book, you will come to see these lies for what they are—attempts to control, manipulate, and imprison you.

My Step-by-Step Program

Throughout the book, I offer you my proprietary step-by-step program, which has proven to be effective for many of my clients throughout the years. This program will help guide you through the process of first recognizing you are being emotionally abused and then deciding whether or not you need to end your relationship. This includes:

- Coming to understand that you are being emotionally abused
- Understanding how emotional abuse is shaming
- Recognizing the damage that emotional abuse and shaming can do to you
- Learning how to stop shaming and blaming yourself and to start seeing your partner more realistically
- Learning how to stop believing the abuser's lies, manipulations, and distortions of reality
- Connecting with and releasing your anger at having been abused.
- Learning how to counter your partner's negative messages by creating an internal nurturing voice
- Learning how to have compassion for your suffering, including ways to comfort yourself and to validate your feelings
- Becoming empowered to stand up for yourself

- Understanding more about your own personal history regarding shame and forgiving yourself for believing the abuser
- Understanding why you stayed so long and forgiving yourself for it
- Continuing to heal your shame

You've taken an important step by choosing this book. There will no doubt be times when you will want to stop reading because the information is so painful, and that's okay. Take your time. In fact, taking your time to absorb the information can be more beneficial than racing through the book, looking for answers. Yes, there is important and powerful information in this book, but the truth is, you may already know some of what I'm sharing with you. You may already have inside you the answers you seek. You may not be in touch with these answers; they may be buried underneath the layers and layers of criticism, lies, and distortions your partner constantly berates you with. But the answers are there nevertheless. Reading slowly, allowing yourself to feel your emotions as you read, will be like diving beneath the layers of confusion, uncertainty, and lies that keep you from seeing your truth.

In addition to important information, I also offer you many exercises and processes to help you find your own truth. Past clients and readers of my other books have shared with me that they have benefited greatly by completing these exercises and processes. For this reason, I encourage you to do the same, preferably as you read the book. This journey is not an easy one, but waiting on the other side is freedom, peace of mind, and a return to the whole and happy person you once were.

CHAPTER 2

Determining Whether You Are Being Emotionally Abused

Before you can break out of prison, you must realize you are locked up.

—ANONYMOUS

SOMETIMES IT'S DIFFICULT TO RECOGNIZE emotional abuse; it's even harder to admit to yourself that, in fact, this is what is happening to you. In this chapter, we will explore why this is so, and I will provide a questionnaire to help you decide.

One of the main reasons why emotional abuse is difficult to recognize is that, unlike physical abuse, with emotional abuse there are no bruises, no outward signs of abuse at all. The wounds are to the heart and the scars are on the mind. Emotional abuse doesn't even always involve words. It can be looks and gestures. Eye-rolling, smirking, frowning, and laughing can all be forms of emotional abuse, especially if done in front of other people. Eventually, an emotional abuser can just look at his partner in a judgmental or mocking way and sigh the familiar sigh of disapproval or frustration. He can roll his eyes in exasperation and look at someone else as if to say, "Oh my God, can you believe she just said that?"

Obstacles in the Way of
Discovering and Facing the Truth

Unfortunately, there are a lot of obstacles in the way of discovering the truth about your situation, but the biggest obstacle is that you probably don't trust your own feelings and your own instincts. In fact, instead of trusting their own instincts, many victims come to believe their partner's accusations and put-downs. For example, if a woman is constantly told that she is lazy, incompetent, and emotionally cold, she will soon come to believe these things about herself. And the irony of the situation is that the more depressed she becomes due to the constant assault on her personality, the less motivated and productive she will become and the less affectionate and sexual she will feel.

My client Ramona's husband constantly complained about her not wanting to have sex with him. "Ever since we got married, you've stop being turned on by me. It's like once you got that ring on your finger, you figured you didn't need to make me happy in bed anymore."

Ramona shared this with me during our first session:

> You know, the truth is, I don't feel attracted to him anymore. I don't know what happened. I used to love having sex with him. But now I don't feel anything for him in that way. I don't blame him for complaining. I wouldn't even blame him for having sex with someone else, the way he always threatens to do. What is wrong with me?

In our work together, Ramona came to realize that her husband's constant faultfinding, unreasonable demands, perfectionism, and possessiveness had caused her to shut down both emotionally and physically. As I explained to her, due to our biological makeup, women need to feel safe and relaxed in order to be receptive to sex. Those who are being constantly put down and emotionally abused will naturally shut down sexually. In other words, our bodies, specifically our genitals, no longer respond by lubricating and relaxing so that sex is comfortable—or even possible. So it was completely understandable that Ramona was no longer interested in sex with her husband. Her body was so shut down that she couldn't have sex without a great deal of pain or discomfort. (Although men's bodies don't respond in the exact same way to abuse, men can emotionally shut down to the point that they no longer feel safe being emotionally vulnerable with their partner.)

Another obstacle in the way of being able to determine whether you are being emotionally abused is the fact that emotional abuse can be very subtle. The following example illustrates some forms of subtle abuse.

My client Tom came into therapy because he was often depressed, was having a difficult time sleeping, and was often sick. He'd been to the doctor for a thorough checkup, and the doctor had given him a clean bill of health but suggested he seek help from counseling. After a few sessions, it became clear that Tom was being emotionally abused.

"My wife is convinced I don't love her, and she looks for evidence of this on a consistent basis. For years, she complained that I never bring her flowers anymore. So a couple of weeks ago, I remembered to stop to buy her flowers on my way home. She took one look at the bouquet and said to me, 'You know I don't like daisies, so why did you buy them?'

"Now, I must confess, she did tell me a long time ago that she didn't like daisies, but I forgot. And when I bought the ready-made bouquet, I didn't even think to ask the florist if it had daisies in it. I guess I should have."

I asked him, "Did your wife acknowledge the fact that you thought of her, that you remembered to bring her flowers?"

"No, she was too upset about the daisies."

"Does it ever feel like you can't win, that you can't ever please her?" I inquired.

"Well, yes, but sometimes I think she's right. Sometimes I doubt that I really love her."

"Why is that?"

"Well, often when I do something to show my love, she accuses me of just playing a role. I tried to make up for the daisies fiasco by taking her out to a really nice place for a romantic dinner. But instead of being happy about it, she looked at me during dinner and said, 'You just want to look good—like you're a good husband. But if you really loved me you wouldn't have bought those daisies.'"

"How did you feel about what she said?"

"Well, it hurt of course, but in a way she was right. I was trying to make up for the mistake I made with the daisies. I wasn't doing it because I was feeling loving."

"And how did you feel about the fact that she brought up the daisies again?" I inquired.

"Well, yes, she does that a lot. She has a hard time letting things go."

Can you see how off balance Tom is, vacillating between admitting how unreasonable his wife is and accepting the blame for the entire situation? Tom readily believes his wife's complaints and accusations. This is because emotional abusers often include just the right amount of truth in their manipulation, enough to confuse and confound their victims.

As you can see from Tom's story, it is not only women who are being emotionally abused. While the most obvious scenario is one in which the man is the emotional abuser and the woman is the victim, there is increasing evidence that men are being emotionally abused almost as much as women. One study that examined intimate partner violence prevalence rates for men and women found men were as likely as women to report perceived emotional abuse. The findings of another study suggest that men's overall risk of emotional abuse may be increasing.

Still another reason why it is so difficult to determine whether you are being emotionally abused is that abusers are very good at deflecting and making excuses for their behavior. When a victim of emotional abuse tries to protest or call her partner on his abusive behavior, she is often accused of "being too sensitive" or "making a big deal out of nothing." Here are some common statements abusive partners make to confuse or disarm their partners:

- "You're overreacting."
- "You're confused. I didn't do that."
- "You're exaggerating. I'm not like that."
- "You misheard me. I would never say that."
- "You have a bad memory. I know what really happened."
- "It's not my fault that you are hypersensitive."
- "You're being overdramatic."
- "I never treat you like that. You're imagining it."
- "You're just being argumentative."
- "You shouldn't let it bother you."
- "You shouldn't think/feel that way."

Did any of the above statements sound familiar to you? If so, make a mental note that these are the kinds of statements that abusive partners use to cause their partners to doubt their feelings and perceptions.

Abusers are also good at distracting and diverting and turning the table on their victims. If you try to tell your partner that he is being too critical, he will likely tell you something like, "*I'm* being critical? That's a laugh. You are the critical one. In fact, that's what you are doing right now!" If you confront your partner about his lying, he'll be quick to point out the last time you lied. (For example, "Aren't you the one who told your sister you were sick to avoid having to go to a family gathering?")

Uncertainty About What Constitutes Emotional Abuse

Still another reason why it is difficult to determine whether you are being emotionally abused is the fact that many people don't know what qualifies as emotional abuse. Throughout this book, I will help you identify exactly what emotional abuse looks, feels, and sounds like so you can distinguish it from the common ways that partners sometimes hurt one another.

When most people think of emotional abuse, they usually think of one partner belittling or criticizing the other. But emotional abuse is much more than verbal abuse. Speaking very broadly, emotional abuse can be defined as *any nonphysical behavior that is designed to control, intimidate, subjugate, demean, punish, or isolate another person through the use of degradation, humiliation, or fear.*

Emotional abuse can include verbal assault, dominance, control, isolation, ridicule, or the use of intimate knowledge for degradation. It targets the emotional and psychological well-being of the victim, and it is often a precursor to physical abuse.

OVERT VERSUS COVERT ABUSE

It is important to note that a pattern of emotional abuse can occur on both an overt and a covert level. *Overt* abuse is openly demeaning. When a wife openly complains to other family members and friends that her husband doesn't make enough money and that he's just too weak to ask for a raise, she is being *overtly* abusive.

Covert emotional abuse is subtler than overt abuse, but no less devastating. When the wife gives her husband contemptuous looks when he tells her they can't afford something and then she offhandedly suggests that maybe some other man might buy it for her, she is being *covertly* abusive.

Emotional abuse is a form of brainwashing that slowly erodes the victims' sense of self-worth, self-confidence, security, and trust in themselves and others. Unlike physical abuse, which often comes out in dramatic outbursts, emotional abuse can be insidious and elusive, slowly disintegrating one's sense of self and personal value.

Emotional abuse can be likened to the slow drip, drip, drip of water torture. The first few drops of water on your forehead don't bother you that much, but soon the constant dripping begins to unnerve you. You spend all your time anticipating when the next drop will come. You become more and more sensitive to the drips until each one feels like a drop of fire on your forehead.

Sometimes emotional abuse occurs suddenly, seemingly out of the blue. The kind and loving person you fell in love with suddenly turns into another person entirely. He becomes critical, impatient, and demanding. The person who loved you so much he couldn't stand to be away from you suddenly can't be in the same room as you without putting you down.

As already noted, emotionally abusive behavior ranges from verbal abuse (belittling, berating, constant criticism) to more subtle tactics (intimidation, manipulation, refusal to be pleased, the silent treatment).

There are also some forms of physical behavior that can be considered emotional abuse. In fact, these behaviors have a name for them—*symbolic violence*. This includes intimidating behavior such as slamming doors; kicking a wall; throwing dishes, furniture, or other objects; driving recklessly while the victim is in the car; and destroying or threatening to destroy objects the victim values. Even milder forms of violence such as shaking a fist or finger at the victim, making threatening gestures or faces, or acting like the abuser wants to kill the victim carry symbolic threats of violence.

Many abusers are so clever and so subtle in their abusive tactics that their abusive behavior can be difficult to identify. Consider my client Jenny's husband, Nathan.

If Jenny asked Nathan to do something, like mow the lawn, he would smile and say, "Sure, I'll do it next Saturday." But when next Saturday came and went, Jenny would notice that the lawn hadn't been mowed. "Why didn't you mow the lawn on Saturday?" she would ask. "Oh, I didn't feel good. I'll do it next weekend" would be his typical response. This scenario would often continue for weeks, with the lawn not being mowed and Nathan making up some excuse for not doing it.

Finally, Jenny began to say, "If you aren't going to mow the lawn, I'll hire someone to do it." At this point, Nathan would blow up. "You are such a nag. I told you I'd get to it. Why do you have to be so controlling?"

This kind of scenario was repeated many times in their marriage. Nathan would agree to bring home milk for their children's cereal the next morning, but he would "forget." He'd "misplace" the car keys when they were going to go to a party he didn't want to go to. He'd "forget" to pick up their kids after a Saturday afternoon movie that he didn't want them to go to in the first place. And if Jenny became angry with him, he became enraged and accused her of being controlling or unreasonable. No matter what Nathan did or didn't do, he never took responsibility for it but instead twisted it around to focus on the fact that Jenny had gotten angry. He was always the victim.

This behavior on her husband's part was what brought Jenny into therapy. "My husband tells me that I'm too impatient and too controlling. But I can't help getting upset when he continually forgets to do things or makes excuses for not doing them. I've gotten to the point where I seldom ask him to do anything. I just do it myself, or I hire someone else to do it. I've stopped asking him to pick up the kids because he's left them waiting too many times. And I constantly feel manipulated by him. When he really doesn't want to do something, instead of just saying he doesn't want to do it, he promises to do it later and then never gets around to it. He accuses me of being controlling, but in reality, he always ends up getting his way. Last night we went to my daughter's favorite restaurant to celebrate her birthday. Even though Nathan says he doesn't like that restaurant, he managed to agree to go for my daughter. Nevertheless, he complained about the food and the service the whole time we were there and ruined our celebration.

"I don't know what to do. I'm so hurt and frustrated by his behavior that I don't want to be around him. But I'm afraid that I am the problem. Maybe I *am* too controlling and impatient; I'm just so confused."

In the process of my working with Jenny, she was able to realize that she was not the controlling one. Nathan was displaying what is called *passive aggressive behavior*. Passive aggressive behaviors are those that involve acting indirectly aggressive rather than directly aggressive. Passive aggressive people regularly exhibit resistance to requests or demands from family and others, often by procrastinating, expressing sullenness, or acting stubborn.

Another aspect of Jenny's husband's behavior that is common among abusive partners is how he managed to turn the tables on Jenny and accuse her of being controlling when, in reality, he was the one with the control issues. As mentioned earlier, this is a common tactic of abusers and is one of the most confusing for the victim. When someone turns the tables on you like this, it causes you to doubt your own perceptions and your own reality.

Facing the Truth

Even when all the signs are there and you recognize how hurtful your partner's behavior is, it can still be difficult to admit you are being emotionally abused. It can be embarrassing to acknowledge that you've allowed yourself to be humiliated, manipulated, demeaned, dismissed, and controlled. It can be particularly embarrassing for men to admit this, but women are often ashamed to admit it as well—especially if they are competent and successful in other areas of their life.

The word *abuse* is itself filled with shame, and in our culture, victims of any kind of abuse have been stigmatized and made to feel that they are weak for putting up with abuse. But being abused is nothing to be ashamed of. And emotional abuse is unfortunately extremely prevalent. Emotional abuse is far more common than physical abuse, and it cuts across all social, economic, racial, and religious lines. While it is hard to determine the exact number of women and men who are emotionally abused worldwide, we know that the number is astronomical. According to one famous study, *35 percent of all women who are or have been in married or common-law relationships have experienced emotional abuse.* Shockingly, new findings from the National Intimate Partner and Sexual Violence Survey state that approximately half of Americans reported experiencing emotional abuse by a partner in a lifetime

Many people who are being emotionally abused tell themselves that their relationship is just going through a rough patch or rationalize that their partner is under a great deal of stress. Or they try to convince themselves that it is "no big deal." Although they may suffer from many of the effects of emotional abuse— such as depression, lack of motivation, confusion, difficulty concentrating or making decisions, low self-esteem, feelings of failure or worthlessness, feelings of hopelessness, self-blame, and self-destructiveness—they do not connect these symptoms with the way their partner is treating them.

Others may not want to face the fact that they are being emotionally abused because it would require them to admit that their relationship has become destructive or force them to face the painful truth about how their partner feels about them. For many, facing the extent of the emotional abuse that has occurred in their relationship would force them to take some action, such as entering marital or individual counseling or even ending the relationship. These actions can be very fear provoking.

Are You Being Emotionally Abused?

To help you identify whether you are being emotionally abused, answer the following questions as honestly as you can.

1. Do you feel you have no voice in your relationship, like you are unimportant?
2. Do you feel like a failure as a partner even though you work hard to please your partner or "get it right"?
3. Do you feel angry, depressed, and anxious because you constantly obsess over trying to solve the problems in the relationship?
4. Does your partner feel you are the one who is responsible for all the problems in the relationship?
5. Does your partner constantly blame or criticize you?
6. Does your partner treat you like a child? Does he constantly correct you or chastise you because your behavior is "inappropriate"?
7. Does your partner need to control all or most aspects of your life? Do you feel you must get permission before going somewhere or before making even the smallest decisions? Do you have to account for any money you spend, or does he attempt to control your spending (even though he has no problem spending on himself)?
8. Have you stopped seeing many or all of your friends and/or family since being in this relationship? Did you do this because your partner dislikes them or feels jealous of the time you spent with them, or because you are ashamed of the way he treats you in front of them?
9. Does your partner treat you as if you are "less than" or inferior to him? Does your partner make a point of reminding you that you are less educated or that you make less money or that you aren't as attractive as he is?

10. Does your partner routinely ridicule, dismiss, or disregard your opinions, thoughts, suggestions, and feelings?

11. Does your partner constantly belittle your accomplishments, your aspirations, or your plans for the future?

12. Do you find yourself "walking on eggshells"? Do you spend a lot of time monitoring your behavior and/or watching for your partner's bad moods before bringing up a subject?

13. Did you stop seeing friends and family because you are ashamed of the fact that you're still with him, even though you've complained to them many times about the way he treats you?

14. Does your partner usually insist on getting his own way? Does he want to be the one to decide where you will go, what you will do, and whom you will do it with?

15. Does your partner punish you by pouting, withdrawing from you, giving you the silent treatment, or withholding affection or sex if you don't do things his way?

16. Does your partner frequently threaten to end the relationship if you don't do things her way?

17. Does your partner constantly accuse you of flirting or of having affairs, even though it isn't true?

18. Does your partner feel she is always right?

19. Does your partner seem impossible to please? Does he constantly complain to you about some aspect of your personality, your looks, or the way you choose to run your life?

20. Does your partner frequently put you down or make fun of you in front of others?

21. Does your partner blame you for his problems? For example, is it your fault he flies off the handle and starts screaming? Does he tell you he wouldn't do it if you didn't make him so mad? Are you to blame for her problem with compulsive overeating? Because he has a

drinking problem? Are you blamed because if he didn't have to support you and the kids, he would have been able to finish college or fulfill his dream of becoming an actor (author, musician, singer, etc.)?

22. Does your partner feel you are the one who is responsible for all the problems in the relationship?

23. Does your partner's personality seem to go through radical changes? Is she pleasant one minute, only to be furious the next? Does he become enraged with only the slightest provocation? Does she experience periods of extreme elation followed by periods of severe depression? Does his personality seem to change when he drinks alcohol?

24. Does your partner tease you, make fun of you, or use sarcasm as a way to put you down or degrade you? Does he especially like to do this in front of others? When you complain, does he tell you that it was just a joke and that you are too sensitive or don't have a sense of humor?

25. Is your partner unable to laugh at herself? Is she extremely sensitive when it comes to others making fun of her or making any kind of comment that seems to show a lack of respect?

26. Does your partner find it difficult or impossible to apologize or admit when he is wrong? Does he make excuses for his behavior or tend to blame others for his mistakes?

27. Does your partner constantly pressure you for sex or try to persuade you to engage in sexual acts that you find repulsive? Has he ever threatened to find someone else who will have sex with him or who will engage in the activities he is interested in?

If you answered yes to even a few of these questions, you are being emotionally abused, and you may be surprised to realize that much of your partner's behavior toward you is actually emotionally abusive. While this is a difficult truth to face, it can also be a liberating one. As the old saying goes, the truth can actually set you free.

Your Reactions to the Questionnaire

Reading the above questions has likely caused you to have some strong emotional reactions. Pay attention to these reactions. For example, how did you feel each time you read a question that described the way your partner treats you? Were you surprised to realize that this behavior is considered emotionally abusive? Or did you feel validated to realize that your suspicion that you were being emotionally abused was accurate?

Did you find that you tended to make excuses for your partner's behavior? Or did you minimize his behavior, telling yourself that "he doesn't do this very often"? It is difficult to admit to yourself that your partner treats you in emotionally abusive ways, so it is understandable that you would make excuses for or minimize his behavior. As you continue reading and doing the exercises I have provided, you will find that it will become easier to admit the truth to yourself.

I want to note that, more than anything else, what characterizes an emotionally abusive relationship is a consistent pattern of hurtful, humiliating, and condescending behavior. For example, if your partner treats you in any of the above ways only rarely, this can be fairly normal. Not healthy, but not necessarily abusive. It is when your partner treats you in any of these above ways on a *consistent basis*, when his abusive behavior becomes more the norm than the exception, that you can confidently say that you are being emotionally abused.

A word of caution: a common quality of many of those who are being abused is to have an odd sense of fairness that can actually get in their way of seeing things clearly. For example, some of you, after looking at the above questionnaire, may resist acknowledging you are being emotionally abused by saying to yourself, "But I am guilty of some of these same behaviors. How can I accuse him of being emotionally abusive if I do the same things?"

Again, focus on the idea of a *pattern of behavior*. We all treat our partners in some of these ways from time to time. No one is perfect. So even if you occasionally treat your partner in some of the above ways, it doesn't mean you are an emotional abuser, especially if your treatment of him is in reaction to his treating you in emotionally abusive ways on a constant basis. I'm not excusing your behavior, but we all tend to treat others the way they treat us. If you occasionally lose your cool after your partner has been barraging you with criticism and you blurt out an insult or criticize him in return, you are not being emotionally abusive. If you sometimes yell at him or call him names in response to his cruelty, you are not an emotional abuser. And if you sometimes refuse to talk to him for hours or days at a time because you feel so wounded that you feel you need to isolate yourself from him to lick your wounds, you are not giving him the silent treatment. Don't let your overblown need to be fair prevent you from seeing what is actually happening in your relationship.

In the next chapter, we will focus on the specific tactics used by emotional abusers. This will help you even further to tell yourself the truth about your relationship and about the way your partner treats you.

CHAPTER 3

Tools of the Trade

Sticks and stones may break our bones, but words will break our hearts.
—ROBERT FULGHUM, *All I Really Need to Know I Learned in Kindergarten*

A s a way to further help clear up any confusion you may still have as to whether you are being emotionally abused, in this chapter I present the most common tactics used by abusive people. The typical emotional abuser has an entire repertoire of tools he or she can use to manipulate and control his or her partner. While not every abuser uses these tactics in a deliberate and conscious way, many do.

The Tactics of Emotional Abuse

Here is an extensive list of all the forms of emotional abuse in alphabetical order. Notice which of the following tactics your partner uses with you.

ABUSIVE EXPECTATIONS: When someone has abusive expectations, they place unreasonable demands on their partner. Expecting you to put everything aside in order to satisfy their needs, demanding your undivided attention, demanding frequent sex, or requiring you to spend all of your time with them are all examples of abusive expectations. This person can *never be pleased* because there is always something more you could have done. You are likely to be subjected to constant criticism and to be berated because you don't fulfill their needs.

This is how my client Susie described her relationship:

> My partner expects me to drop everything I'm doing as soon as she comes home and to give her my undivided attention. I work from home, so sometimes I'm right in the middle of something important, but that doesn't matter. She sits down, gets a drink, and starts to tell me all about her day. I'm supposed to sit there and listen attentively no matter how long she goes on. The more she drinks, the longer she talks. Sometimes I feel like a prisoner because I know what would happen if I tell her I need to get up because I have to do something. She'd go into a tirade about how I don't love her, how I'm not interested in her life, etcetera, etcetera. God forbid if I want to tell her about my day. There's no such thing as a two-way street in this relationship. It is clearly all about her.

CHARACTER ASSASSINATION: This involves constantly blowing someone's mistakes out of proportion; humiliating, criticizing, or making fun of someone in front of others; or discounting another person's achievements. It can also include lying about someone in order to negatively affect others' opinion of that person or gossiping about a person's failures and mistakes with others. In addition to the pain this behavior can cause an individual on a personal level, character assassination also can ruin someone's personal and professional reputation, causing that person to lose friends, jobs, or even their family.

This is exactly what happened with my client Avery:

My husband is very insecure and threatened by the attention I get from men. He hated it when I went out with my girlfriends, even if it was just for dinner. He was convinced I was always flirting with other men, although this was the furthest thing from my mind. I just wanted to connect with someone other than him and have a good time. Eventually, he became convinced I was cheating on him with another man. He even went so far as telling my family I was having an affair with someone. He got close to my parents, and whenever I went out with my friends he'd go see them and tell them his sob story about how much he loved me and how I was breaking his heart by being unfaithful. My parents felt sorry for him, and my mother even took me to lunch one day to beg me to not break up my marriage because of this affair. No matter how much I tried to make her understand that I wasn't having an affair, it didn't do any good. My husband had convinced her I was.

My husband also complained to my sister and her husband, and they also believed him. And because they are very religious, my sister told me that unless I ended my affair they had to stop seeing me. This was devastating to me, not only because I was close to my sister, but I love my niece and nephew dearly, and my sister didn't allow me to see them because she didn't want me to be a negative influence on them.

CONSTANT CHAOS/CREATING CRISES: Specifically characterized by continual upheavals and discord, this type of behavior will cause you to feel constantly unsettled and off-balance. If your partner deliberately starts arguments with you or others or seems to be in constant conflict with others, he or she may be "addicted to drama." Creating drama or chaos provides excitement for some people, especially those who distract themselves from their problems by focusing outward, those who feel empty inside and need to fill themselves up with activity, and those who were raised in an environment in which harmony and peace were unknown quantities. Constant chaos can also be a reflection of what is going on inside of a person and is characteristic of borderline personality disorder, which we will discuss in later chapters when we discuss the different types of abusive partners.

As my client Aaron explained to me, life was never calm around his wife, Sherry. "She's always starting trouble. I don't think I can remember one day since I've known her when she wasn't fighting with someone. If she's not angry with someone at work, she's arguing with one of her sisters or her mother. Everything seems like a big deal to her, and she can't ever just let something go. I have to hear about it over and over. And I never know what to expect when I come home. She might be in a good mood and we have a good evening, or she might be angry at me for something and I'm in for a rough night." While Aaron was initially attracted to Sherry's drama, it was beginning to take a toll on him. "I don't sleep well at night, and I'm always nervous. I've lost my appetite, and I keep losing weight. And I know all this drama and chaos isn't good for the kids."

CONSTANT CRITICISM: Constant criticism can be a form of verbal assault. It is when your partner constantly points out your mistakes, flaws, or shortcomings. This is often done under the guise of trying to "help" you or "guide" you toward being a better person, but make no mistake, the purpose of constant criticism is to shame you and make you doubt yourself or feel bad about yourself so he or she can control and/or manipulate you into doing his or her bidding.

It is the insidious nature and cumulative effect of this type of abuse that does the damage. Over time, it eats away at your self-confidence and sense of self-worth, undermining any good feelings you have about yourself and about your accomplishments.

When a partner overtly criticizes or screams and yells, it is easy to come to the conclusion that you are being emotionally abused, but when your partner puts you down under the guise of humor, it can be extremely difficult to come to this realization. In my client Steve's case, it took a friend calling it to his attention before he realized his wife was emotionally and verbally abusing him with constant criticism.

Steve's wife, Nancy, was a fun-loving woman who laughed and joked a lot. She loved to socialize and was always the life of the party. Steve was a rather quiet man, and he found Nancy's ease with people refreshing and stimulating. He often told her he wished he could be more like her. So when Nancy began to tease him about being "socially retarded" right after they got married, Steve just laughed right along with her. But this was only the beginning. Nancy began to make jokes about Steve in front of others: "Please excuse Steve. He forgot to wake up this morning." Steve took this as a gentle reminder that he needed to participate more in conversations, and he forced himself to talk about himself and his interests when they had company. But whenever he did this, Nancy would feign a yawn or roll her eyes, signaling to him that he was being boring. Steve would take the hint and go back into his shell. He decided he was better off being a listener and letting Nancy be the socializer.

But Nancy didn't stop there. She started in on the way he dressed, the way he carried himself, and his general demeanor. She called him the "Professor"—teasing him about how conservatively he dressed. "Don't you have even one tie with some color to it?" or "How long have you had that suit anyway?" she'd complain when they were going out. "Stand up straight," she'd order. "You look like a tired old man." Most of the time Steve just tried to laugh off Nancy's comments, even though he was sometimes deeply hurt by them. Often, he took her seriously, and believing that Nancy was just looking out for him, he actually made some changes, such as improving his posture and buying some new, more stylish clothes. If anyone would have told Steve that he was being emotionally abused, he would have told them they were crazy. After all, Nancy was just trying to help him out.

It wasn't until his best friend, Larry, came to visit him from back East that Steve began to recognize he was being emotionally abused. "Larry was shocked at how Nancy talked to me," Steve told me during one of our sessions. "And he was surprised to see me just taking it instead of standing up for myself. He told me I'd gone from a self-assured, congenial kind of guy to an insecure, withdrawn man he barely recognized. He asked me why I let her talk to me that way. When I tried to explain it was just her sense of humor, he said, 'Bullshit, she's putting you down all the time.' I finally had to admit he was right."

CONTINUAL BLAMING: This is when your partner blames you for anything that goes wrong. It is always your fault; you are always doing something wrong, always disappointing her, always showing her that you don't love her.

This is how my client Walter described his situation:

> If my wife does poorly at work, she finds a way to blame me. If she isn't getting along with her mother, she blames me. If she gains weight, she blames me. As far as she is concerned, I am to blame for everything bad that happens to her.
>
> For a long time, I believed her. I didn't recognize that she can never take responsibility for any of her actions. I already had low self-esteem when I got married, so it came naturally for me to blame myself. But I've been reading a lot of books, and I've come to realize that this is my wife's problem, not mine. She has even lower self-esteem than I do, and she can't handle failure of any kind, so she immediately puts the blame on someone else, usually me.

CONTROLLING BEHAVIOR: Controlling behavior is just what it sounds like. Your partner has a need to control every aspect of your life: your finances, how you discipline your children, even what you wear. He may treat you like a child who needs to be managed and controlled. He doesn't see you as an equal partner, but as someone who is not as smart or competent as he is. He may even require that you get his permission before you can go anywhere or make any major decisions.

DOMINATION: Someone who needs to dominate in a relationship has a tremendous need to have his or her own way and often resorts to threats in order to get it. Domineering behavior includes: ordering a partner around; monitoring time and activities; restricting resources (finances, telephone); restricting social activities; isolating a partner from her family or friends; interfering with opportunities (job, education, medical care); showing excessive jealousy and possessiveness; throwing objects; threatening to or harming a partner or a partner's children, family, friends, pets, or property; and forcing or coercing a partner into illegal activity.

I met Paula at a battered women's center where I used to volunteer. Paula came from a deeply religious family in which she was expected to obey her father without question, so she didn't think anything about it when her husband insisted on controlling everything in their relationship—their finances, their sex life, even her daily schedule. This is how she explained it to me.

> He didn't want me to work, so I became a housewife. But don't think I had it easy. I had to keep the house immaculate. He actually went around checking to see if there was dust on the furniture or if the floors were dirty. He even wrote up a schedule of what I should do every week. Laundry on Monday, shopping for groceries on Tuesday and Friday. And, of course, he

wrote up a shopping list and dictated what I should cook every day.

This went on for a couple of years. Although I wasn't happy, I didn't realize anything was terribly wrong. That is, until I had our daughter, Mary. Then my husband became impossible with his demands. He insisted the baby only wear cotton diapers instead of Pampers. When the baby cried, he insisted I let her cry so she wouldn't become spoiled. He demanded she become potty-trained way before she was ready; he even forced her to sit on the toilet when she could hardly sit up.

This is where I drew the line. I had been willing to follow all his rules no matter how ridiculous they were when it was just the two of us. But I couldn't stand what he was doing to Mary. She was not a happy child, and I knew it was because she wasn't allowed to just be a child—to play and be free.

I knew he wasn't going to change, and I didn't want my child to be dominated by her father the way he dominated me. So I decided I needed to leave and take Mary with me. I knew he wouldn't let me go, so I had to run away when he wasn't home and come here.

EMOTIONAL BLACKMAIL: Emotional blackmail is one of the most powerful forms of manipulation. It occurs when one partner either consciously or unconsciously coerces the other into doing what he wants by playing on his partner's fear, guilt, or compassion. Examples of emotional blackmail include one partner threatening to end the relationship if he doesn't get what he wants or one partner rejecting or distancing herself from her partner until he gives into her demands. If your partner withholds sex or affection or gives you the silent treatment or the cold shoulder whenever he is displeased with you, threatens to find someone else, or uses other fear tactics to get you under control, he is using the tactic of emotional blackmail.

Threats of emotional blackmail don't have to be overt. In fact, they are often quite subtle. For example, a woman may jokingly suggest that her boyfriend better start paying more attention to her sexually if he wants to keep her. Or, in order to get his wife to do as he wishes, a man may threaten her by saying that it will be difficult to find a new partner who is willing to get involved with a woman who already has two children. Those who use the tactic of emotional blackmail also use guilt in order to get their way or keep their partner in line. This was the case with my client Rubin. Rubin's wife didn't like to be alone. She especially hated it when he had to go out of town on business.

> Whenever I had to take a trip, she'd beg me not to go. I'd try to explain to her that I had to go, that I'd lose my job if I didn't. But she'd argue with me that if I really loved her I would look for another job, one that didn't require travel. When I went out the door the morning of a trip, she'd look at me like a wounded child. I felt horribly guilty leaving her all alone.
>
> I'd leave anyway, but I felt terrible about doing it. I'd call her every night, and she'd cry on the phone for me to please come home. It ripped my heart out. And to make matters worse, almost every time I took a trip, she ended up getting sick. Sometimes she'd get so sick she'd end up in the hospital. I'd have to cut my trip short to come home to her.
>
> It wasn't like she faked getting sick; she really got sick. But she also got miraculously better as soon as I was back. I finally got so tired of feeling guilty that I quit my job and found one that didn't require travel. But the problem is, it pays only about half as much as the other job, and now we are really struggling financially.

The following are warning signs that you are being emotionally blackmailed:

- Your partner asks you to choose between something you want to do and him.
- Your partner tries to make you feel like you are selfish or a bad person if you do something he doesn't want you to do.
- Your partner asks you to give up something or someone as a way of proving your love for him.
- Your partner threatens to leave you if you don't change.
- Your partner threatens to withhold money or access to money unless you do something he has requested.

GASLIGHTING: When someone intentionally twists your perception of reality for their own gain, they are gaslighting you. The term comes from the classic 1944 movie *Gaslight*, in which a husband uses a variety of insidious techniques to make his wife doubt her perceptions, her memory, and her very sanity in order to make her and others believe she is insane. For instance, he keeps dimming the lights in their home (which were powered by gas). When his wife points out that the lights had dimmed, he denies that the lights had changed. His motive was to gain access to her substantial wealth. Gaslighting is sometimes used by those who need to discredit their partner in order to get access to their money or in order to turn others against them.

A partner who gaslights may continually deny that certain events occurred or that he or she said something you both know was said, or he or she may insinuate that you are exaggerating or lying. In this way, the abusive person may be trying to gain control over you or to avoid taking responsibility for his or her actions. This is one of the forms of emotional abuse that is done very consciously and deliberately. It is often used as a way to justify the abuser's own inappropriate, cruel, or abusive behavior.

Gaslighting tends to happen very gradually. The abuser's actions may seem like just harmless misunderstandings at first. Over time, however, these abusive behaviors continue, and a victim can become confused, anxious, disoriented, isolated, and depressed, eventually losing all sense of what is actually happening. Then, the victim may start relying on the abusive partner more and more to define reality, which creates a very difficult situation to escape from.

"Sometimes I think I'm crazy," my client Becky shared with me.

> My husband tells me he loves me, and I really have no reason to doubt him, and yet it often seems to me that he deliberately tries to make me doubt myself. For example, I'll see him flirting with a woman at a party, but when I confront him with it he swears it isn't true. He'll say I'm just imagining things because I'm so insecure, and he'll remind me that he's a friendly guy to everyone. I start telling myself that it is true, I am insecure, and that he is a friendly person, and pretty soon I start to think I must have imagined the whole thing after all. Is this common? Do people really imagine they are seeing things when it isn't really happening?

Although in rare cases people do imagine seeing things that aren't happening, in Becky's case it turned out that her husband had been having numerous affairs during their marriage and that he used gaslighting techniques to keep her confused and off-balance.

INVASION OF PRIVACY: This behavior is actually common among many abusers, but there are some who carry this behavior to extremes. My client Todd's husband is a good example.

> My husband thinks he has the right to look inside my briefcase, my drawers—anything I own. He opens my

mail, listens in on my phone calls, and breaks into my
e-mail account. When I call him on this behavior, he becomes defensive and accuses me of hiding something.
"If you're not doing anything wrong, it shouldn't bother
you so much," he'll say. When we were first married, I
bought this logic, thinking that we were, in fact, married and what was mine was his, and so forth, but as
time has gone by, I began to see it for what it is. He has
a need to do this so he can control me.

Another form of invasion of privacy involves boundary cross-
ing. My client Gloria shared with me how her husband constantly
invades her privacy by barging into the bathroom when she is in
there, even when she is on the toilet or in the shower.

I want to lock the bathroom door, but he has convinced me that since we only have one bathroom it
isn't fair to keep him out. But he often comes in just
to tell me something, not because he has to use the
facilities.

He has the same lack of respect for my body. He
constantly grabs my breasts or butt when he passes by
me, even though I've told him a million times that I
hate it. He just laughs and says, "I can't help it, you're
just so juicy." He seems to be oblivious to how uncomfortable I am with his intrusions. I feel like I have no
space, no privacy, and that I'm constantly being invaded. It is very unsettling. I find that I'm increasingly
nervous and tense all the time, just waiting for the next
invasion.

Invasion of privacy is one of the forms of emotional abuse that
isn't necessarily done in order to control or manipulate the other
person, but whether it is deliberate or not, it can be extremely

shaming. As we will discuss in the next chapter, being shamed can cause us to feel *exposed* and *humiliated.*

ISOLATING BEHAVIOR: Emotional abusers know that if they can isolate you from other people they can gain more control over you and affect your thinking and behavior. Isolating you from others is a way to undermine your life and identity outside of the relationship and foster a sense of dependency. Therefore, they often begin by telling you such things as your family doesn't support you, a particular friend isn't to be trusted, and so on. Eventually, an abusive partner may even refuse to allow you to see family members or friends.

Younger women may be more vulnerable to isolation within their relationships because they may put a higher value on emotional connectivity than independence, and younger women may value a romantic partnership more than the benefits of life as a single person.

Anita's boyfriend, Carl, felt threatened by her close relationship with her parents. He told her in the beginning of their relationship that he didn't want them "interfering" with their relationship, so he refused to let her see them very often or even to talk on the phone with them. If her mother called, Carl would always insist that Anita hang up after only a few minutes because he needed her for something, or he'd make so much noise in the background that she couldn't hear what her mother was saying.

JEKYLL-AND-HYDE SYNDROME: As I wrote in my book *The Jekyll and Hyde Syndrome,* we all experience mood shifts from time to time. We are all multifaceted people who show different sides of ourselves depending on the circumstances and whom we are associating with. And we are all sometimes shocked by our own actions or by the words that come out of our mouths.

But there are some people whose mood shifts are far from normal—people who experience radical changes in their moods and

violent outbursts for no apparent reason, people who become enraged, abusive, or violent at the drop of a hat. There are people
who not only show a different side of themselves depending on the
circumstances and who they are around, but who also are capable
of creating a double life or an entirely different personality—a personality that would be unrecognizable to people who know them
in another context. Those who have a partner with this syndrome
suffer from incredible pain, fear, chaos, and confusion.

The Dr. Jekyll/Mr. Hyde syndrome is named after the classic
Robert Louis Stevenson story "The Strange Case of Dr. Jekyll and
Mr. Hyde," about an upstanding, teetotaling philanthropic doctor
who turns into a womanizing, drinking, scoundrel—seemingly
overnight. The book is a metaphor for a phenomenon that is all too
common: the fact that so-called good people often have a dark side,
a part of themselves they keep hidden from themselves and others.
In some cases, this dark side actually forms a distinct personality
that is radically different from their public persona. Ironically, it is
often those who stand out as the most moral, the most kind, and
the most magnanimous who are the most likely to fall. It seems to
be a rule of nature that the higher up on a pedestal we put ourselves or allow others to put us, the farther we have to fall.

While Dr. Jekyll completed his transformation in the darkness
of night, with no one else witnessing his change, those with the
Dr. Jekyll/Mr. Hyde syndrome often change their personality or
experience their mood shifts in front of others. For example, a
typically loving, patient mother can suddenly burst into a rage, calling her children horrible names, throwing objects across the
room, even driving off without them to teach them a lesson. A
normally pleasant, amiable person can suddenly turn into an insulting, abusive maniac whenever someone crosses him.

Jennifer devotes her life to her husband and children. She is a
stay-at-home mom who is usually patient and loving with her children, four-year-old Erin and six-year-old Josh. But sometimes, for
no apparent reason, Jennifer becomes very impatient and critical

of her kids and husband. Nothing they can do will please her. It is as if she is looking at them through different eyes. The qualities she complimented them on just days before seem to have completely slipped her mind, and all she can see are their faults. "It's all or nothing with my wife," her husband, Bill, told me when, out of desperation, he came to me for help. "You're either the greatest person she ever met or the worst. I've learned to just lay low and wait for her to switch back. But I don't want my kids to have to grow up this way."

Often, a person with this syndrome changes his or her personality depending on whether he or she is in public or in private. For example, the model employee who is affable and cooperative at the office can become a demanding, critical, and verbally abusive father and husband when he comes home. His boss and co-workers would never imagine that the man they know at work could behave in such a way. On the other hand, his wife and children would be shocked to see their demanding father subjugating himself before his boss and laughing with coworkers.

From my many years of experience working as a psychotherapist specializing in abuse, I have determined that there are five distinct types of Dr. Jekyll/Mr. Hydes, including:

1. **The person who is "triggered" by past events (usually childhood trauma):** This person may act perfectly normal in most situations, but when she is reminded of previous trauma, she changes radically, often taking on a completely different personality and often reenacting the type of abuse she herself experienced. This type of person is highly unpredictable. Things can be going along just fine, and suddenly she becomes enraged and blows up at those around her. She usually does not know what set her off, nor do those around her.

2. **The classic Dr. Jekyll/Mr. Hyde who truly lives a double life:** This person may be one person around his

family and an entirely different one when he is away from them. Or he may appear to the public to be the pinnacle of virtue, while at home he abuses his wife and children.

3. **The person whose personality radically changes when he drinks alcohol, takes drugs, or engages in other addictive activities:** Like Dr. Jekyll, whose transformation occurred after taking an elixir he created in his laboratory, this type of radical shift usually takes place only when the person is "altered" due to alcohol, drugs, gambling, and other addictive behaviors.

4. **The person whose opinion of others fluctuates drastically:** This person tends to either view someone as "all good" or "all bad." When she views someone as all bad, she feels justified in treating that person very poorly.

5. **The person who changes dramatically when you challenge him in any way:** This person is kind, considerate, and agreeable as long as things are going his way. But if you don't do as he wants, if you challenge him in any way or if you dare contradict him, you will see a completely different person. He will become defensive, insulting, and cruel.

This transformation is not a normal shift in moods. The aspects that set someone with a Dr. Jekyll/Mr. Hyde syndrome apart are:

- The fact that their mood shifts are far more severe than the average person's.
- In many cases, not only do their moods shift but their entire personality also changes.
- Those with this syndrome seldom own up to or admit to their dual personality or severe mood shifts. In fact, some are not aware that they have such extreme mood shifts or that they have two distinctive personalities.

- Their personality changes often represent a deep conflict within themselves (e.g., the minister who is very much against adultery but has strong sexual urges he cannot control).
- Their personality shifts or dual personalities are often symptomatic of a personality disorder or are due to previous abuse experiences. (Many of those who suffer from the Dr. Jekyll/Mr. Hyde syndrome were abused in childhood, and many suffer from a personality disorder because of it.)

OVERLY JEALOUS, POSSESSIVE BEHAVIOR, INCLUDING STALKING: No matter how innocent or platonic a relationship might be with a friend, coworker, or even a family member, your partner has a way of twisting it into something sordid, selfish, or wrong. She acts out with jealous tantrums or accusatory questions, and no matter what you say, no matter how much you try to explain, she isn't having it. She is so convinced that her perceptions are correct that there is no opening for the truth. The more you try to explain, the more she can make you look guilty, so it usually isn't worth trying.

This is what my client Claire told me about her situation:

> "My husband is insanely jealous. He accuses me of flirting if I even look at another man. I've gotten so I make sure my eyes are fixed on him when we are out just so I don't give him anything to accuse me of.
>
> If a man calls the house asking for me, he interrogates the guy, asking him who he is, how he knows me, and what he wants from me. Even after he does this, he still creates an entire scenario in his mind about who the man is. He constantly tells me that he has great instincts and that he "knows" when I am cheating.
>
> Actually, he couldn't be further from the truth. I love my husband, and I am extremely attracted to him.

I let him know this in every way I can. But he is so insecure that nothing I do assures him that I'm not cheating.

He sometimes goes to the extreme of following me
to see if I'm meeting a man for lunch, and at least once
he traveled all the way to another city to spy on me at
a business conference.

I've tried to be understanding about his insecurities,
but instead of getting better with time, he is actually getting worse. It feels to me like his suspicions are verging
on paranoia. I'm getting to the point that I can't tolerate
his constant accusations. I know I'm a good wife, but
I'm beginning to feel hopeless and helpless about things
changing. I don't think I can go on this way.

PASSIVE-AGGRESSIVE BEHAVIOR: Procrastination is the primary way
people exhibit passive-aggressive behavior. Because they really
don't want to do something or go somewhere, they will find excuses for putting it off. If they are forced to complete a task, they
will wait until the very last second in order to punish the person
who assigned the task. Passive-aggressive behavior may manifest
itself in a number of other ways as well, including sulking when
they don't get their way, offering backhanded compliments, withdrawing and refusing to communicate (silent treatment), and
making excuses to avoid certain people as a way of expressing
their dislike or anger toward those individuals. Ignoring requests
entirely can also be a passive-aggressive action.

The reason passive-aggressive behavior can be emotionally
abusive is that it can cause you to believe that you are too demanding, controlling, or impatient. Because your partner acts in
an agreeable way and doesn't overtly express his anger at being
asked to do something, you may also end up feeling guilty when
you get angry at him for not doing what he said he would do. Any
behavior on your partner's part that causes you to doubt your perceptions or question who you are can be emotionally abusive, and

passive-aggressive behavior is at the top of the list, right along with gaslighting.

SEXUAL HARASSMENT: Normally, the term *sexual harassment* is used to refer to sexual coercion in the workplace, but a person can be sexually harassed by anyone, including her partner. Sexual harassment is defined as unwelcome sexual advances or physical or verbal conduct of a sexual nature. Whenever a person is pressured into becoming sexual against her will, whether it is because she does not feel like being sexual at the time or does not want to engage in a particular sexual act, it is sexual harassment. It is sexual harassment to try to force a partner into engaging in sexual acts that she has no interest in or that upset or repulse her. Oftentimes, other forms of emotional abuse go hand in hand with sexual harassment, such as unreasonable expectations, constant criticism, name-calling, and emotional blackmail.

Eileen's husband, Sam, constantly pressured her to have sex. He expected sex every night and every morning and would sometimes wake up in the middle of the night with an erection and start nudging her in the behind with it. Not only were his sexual demands considered to be sexual harassment, but they were also a form of unreasonable expectations because even when Eileen complied, he never seemed to be happy. "He'd complain that I didn't get into it enough or that I didn't move the right way."

Eileen believed that it was her wifely duty to have sex with her husband whenever he wanted it, and she was afraid he'd go elsewhere for sex if she didn't comply. In fact, he used this as a form of emotional blackmail by telling her, "If you don't do it, I'll find someone else who will."

Sam also pressured Eileen to engage in all kinds of "kinky" sex acts, many of which repulsed her. When she refused, he'd threaten to find someone who would agree to do the things he wanted to do. This emotional blackmail almost always worked since Eileen was horribly afraid of losing him. "I know it sounds ridiculous, but as much as I hate all the sexual pressure, I'd hate it even more if he actually went through with it and had sex with someone else. I'd feel like such a failure, like I couldn't even satisfy my own husband."

SILENT TREATMENT: This occurs primarily when your partner punishes you with silence if he doesn't get his way. This silence may last hours or even days.

The silent treatment may be your partner's way of telling you that you have done something wrong. As a consequence, he refuses to communicate with you or acknowledge you or enter into any form of meaningful dialog with you. He may become emotionally detached and distance himself from you by ignoring your very existence. He may go so far as to avoid eye contact or stare straight through you, making you feel invisible or insignificant. It can include prolonged periods of not only silence but also unresponsiveness. He can even go so far as to exclude you from his life and withhold information, making you feel like an outsider, a form of silent treatment known as "stonewalling."

It's unreasonable to expect you to interpret your partner's silence. Nevertheless, you may find yourself taking on the role of the peacemaker, continually reaching out and trying to make amends. You may apologize profusely in order to get your partner to begin talking to you again. You may begin to feel so insecure in your relationship that you develop a fear of abandonment. And this constant state of apologizing and assuming guilt can greatly diminish your ability to develop and cultivate a healthy sense of self-worth.

In addition to causing you distress, being ignored and excluded can be very shaming. It can threaten your basic psychological need for belonging. By punishing you with the silent treatment, your partner is attempting to induce feelings of powerlessness and shame.

One type of emotional abuser, *the narcissist*, tends to use stonewalling more than other types. While many people think of narcissists as having huge egos and extremely high self-esteem, in actuality, their so-called self-confidence and bravado mask a very fragile ego. Because of this, they tend to demand to be worshipped and adored, and they become enraged if you challenge their authority or if you disrespect them in some way. As a result, they can become emotionally withholding as a way of punishing you and keeping you in your place.

Your desire to keep the peace or work through any conflict helps put a narcissist right back where he wants to be—in control. The more you reach out to him, the more self-righteous he becomes. He will maintain his silence until he feels you have been sufficiently punished. He knows that by ignoring you, he is devaluing your very existence and making you feel insignificant.

SYMBOLIC VIOLENCE: As stated earlier, although emotional abuse usually includes only nonphysical forms of abuse, it can include what is called symbolic violence: gestures (e.g., pointing a finger in your face, making a fist) and actions (e.g., throwing things, breaking something you love) that are intended to frighten you and control you.

THREATENING BEHAVIOR: This includes making subtle and not-so-subtle threats or negative remarks with the intent to frighten or control you. It can also include threatening divorce whenever you have an argument or threatening infidelity if you don't give in to his sexual demands.

UNDERMINING AND SABOTAGING YOUR EFFORTS: This can be a form of passive-aggressive behavior since there is the same sense of underhandedness to it. A good example of this form of emotional abuse is when you want to do something or go somewhere and your partner acts as if he's okay with it. He may even act enthusiastic while all along he disapproves of it. This was the situation with my client Naomi:

When I told my husband I wanted to go back to school, he seemed all for it. He even asked me if there was anything he could do to support me. I told him that it would be really helpful if he watched the kids on the nights I had classes, and he agreed to do it. But once school started, his offer to be helpful seemed to go right out the window. Instead of watching the kids on my nights to go to school, he started coming home late from work. Since he wasn't there to watch the kids and I didn't feel comfortable leaving them alone, I'd have to scramble around to try to find someone to babysit. Several nights, I couldn't find anyone at the last minute, so I had to miss class. When I called him on it, he got defensive and told me he couldn't help it if his boss asked him to stay late. When I mentioned that he could have called me, he got upset and told me I was attacking him.

When I decided to hire a regular babysitter, my husband complained about how much school was costing us. He told me, "Between the cost of your classes and books and now babysitting, this is becoming a costly venture. What good is it to take these classes? It's not like they are going to help you get a job or anything." I realized then and there that he had never wanted me to go back to school in the first place.

UNPREDICTABLE RESPONSES: This type of emotional abuse includes drastic mood swings and sudden emotional outbursts for no apparent reason, including screaming, cursing, crying jags, and throwing things. It can also include inconsistent responses, such as reacting very differently at various times to the same behavior. For example, he may say one thing one day and the opposite the next, or he may frequently change his mind—liking something one day but hating it the next.

This was my client Patty's experience:

> Last week when I made my pot roast, my husband told
> me he loved it. This week when I made it, he refused to
> eat it, telling me he hates pot roast before storming out
> of the house.

The reason this behavior is damaging is that it causes others, especially a partner, to feel constantly on edge. You are always waiting for the other shoe to drop, and you never feel you know what is expected of you. Living with someone who is like this is extremely demanding and anxiety provoking, causing you to feel constantly frightened, unsettled, and off-balance and to feel that you must remain hypervigilant, waiting for your partner's next outburst or change of mood.

This type of abusive behavior can be an indication of mental illnesses such as bi-polar disorder or of certain personality disorders such as borderline personality disorder.

Using Your Secrets Against You: When we first begin a relationship, we often open up and tell our new partner very intimate, embarrassing things about ourselves, including information about our history or our family's history. This is a natural part of becoming close to someone. But some emotional abusers will use this intimate information against us as a way of humiliating us, whether in the midst of an argument or as a reminder that they could use the information against us by sharing it with others. This kind of emotional abuse actually has a name: the use of intimate knowledge for degradation.

Verbal Assault: This is a particularly potent form of emotional abuse that can include all of the following:

- Swearing at you or calling you names
- Using sarcasm or so-called teasing to put you down or make you feel bad

· Making jokes at your expense, often in front of others
· Ordering you around and treating you like a servant

Verbal assault includes berating, belittling, humiliating, name-calling, screaming, threatening, excessive blaming, shaming, using sarcasm in a cutting way, and expressing disgust toward a person. This kind of abuse is extremely damaging to a person's self-esteem and self-image. Just as assuredly as physical violence assaults the body, verbal abuse assaults the mind and spirit, causing wounds that are extremely difficult to heal. Yelling and screaming are not only demeaning but frightening as well. When someone yells at us, we become afraid that he or she may also resort to physical violence.

I first began seeing Robert and Catherine in couple's counseling. Robert reported that he was constantly exasperated with his wife, Catherine. "I just can't believe you could have been so stupid" was one of his typical phrases. Others included "Get your head out of your butt" and "What were you thinking?" The insinuation was always the same—that Catherine wasn't very smart.

These comments started shortly after Catherine and Robert were married. "I do make a lot of mistakes," Catherine explained to me. "I don't blame him for getting impatient with me." Catherine didn't seem to understand that Robert's comments were hurting her emotionally and that his constant chastising was damaging her self-esteem. "I try to hide my mistakes from him because I know he's going to tell me how stupid I am when if he finds out," Catherine finally admitted. And she admitted something else as well. "When I'm around Robert I seem to make more mistakes than usual. I guess it's because I'm so worried I'll goof up that I end up doing just that."

Both Robert and Catherine seemed to feel that he had the right to chastise her and call her names, even after I explained to both of them that Robert was actually verbally abusing Catherine. Robert quit therapy shortly afterward, but I continued to see

Catherine. As time went on, Robert became more and more abusive and Catherine began to feel more and more inadequate. One day, she broke down and started sobbing as she told me something particularly cruel that Robert had said. This was the turning point for Catherine. She finally recognized she was being abused and how it was damaging her.

WITHHOLDING (RESOURCES, AFFECTION): This type of emotional abuse can go hand in hand with the silent treatment. The purpose is to punish you. Your partner may withhold affection, sex, money, or other "privileges" in an attempt to control you and get his way.

YOU MAY BE surprised to realize that many of the behaviors you live with every day are actually considered emotionally abusive. And even though you may not have labeled these negative and upsetting behaviors as abusive, they have nevertheless hurt you and even damaged you in many ways. Or you may feel validated as you realize that your sense that your partner's behavior is abusive was absolutely correct. No matter how much your partner justifies his behavior, there is no justification for insensitivity, spitefulness, and cruelty.

ALL THE WAYS YOU ARE BEING EMOTIONALLY ABUSED

- Using the above comprehensive list as a reference, make a list of all the ways you are being emotionally abused.
- Now read over your list and take in what you've written down. Take a deep breath and say the words, "I'm being emotionally abused in all these ways." If you can't say the words out loud, say them silently to yourself.

Notice how you feel when you say these words. Some people are afraid to say the words, "I'm being emotionally abused," even to themselves. If this is your situation, notice why you are feeling so afraid. Does it feel like someone is going to come around the corner and smack you if you say these words? Do you feel that just by saying these words to yourself you are being disloyal to your partner? Do you feel that now that you've said these words, you have to do something about the abuse? Do you feel relieved now that you've finally said them? If so, say them again: "I'm being emotionally abused in all these ways." Feel the power in those words, the strength. Acknowledge the courage it takes to say them. Now say the words out loud: "I'm being emotionally abused in all these ways." You may feel sad to admit that you are being emotionally abused. If so, let yourself feel this sadness. It is terribly sad to realize this. Let yourself cry if you need to.

Some of you may notice that you feel angry after saying the words "I'm being emotionally abused in all these ways." If this is your situation, allow yourself to feel and express this anger. Find a safe way to express your righteous anger by doing one or all three of the following:

1. Write a letter to your partner telling him exactly how you feel about his abusive treatment of you. You can decide later if you actually want to give your partner the letter.
2. Imagine that you are talking directly to your partner. Tell her how you feel about the fact that you have been abused by her. Don't hold back and don't censor yourself. Say everything that comes to mind. You can use swear words, you can blame and accuse. There's no wrong way to express this anger.
3. Find a physical way to express your anger. Ask your body how it would like to express the anger. Some

people need to release their anger by shouting, others want to throw something, and still others want to break things or tear things up. Do whatever your body wants to do to release the anger stored in your body.

Honor whatever response you had to this exercise. Whatever you feel is okay. Keep your list in a place where your partner will be unable to find it, and refer to it as you continue to read this book. It can become the reminder you need when you are confused, the validation you seek when you question whether you are being abused.

How Has Emotional Abuse Affected You?

After you have taken some time to absorb the fact that you are being emotionally abused in all the ways you have listed, it is time to focus on the effects this abuse has had on you. We will discuss the primary damage that emotionally abusive behavior has on a person in the next two chapters, focusing on shame in particular, but for now, take some time to consider how you have been wounded and damaged by your partner's emotional abuse. If you feel stuck, refer back to the list of effects on pages 18–19.

You may wish to start by writing down this sentence:

"I've been wounded by my partner's emotional abuse in the following ways:

Or it can also help to complete the following sentences:

"The emotional abuse from my partner has caused me to

_____ ."

"I am less _____ due to the way my partner treats me."

"I am more _____ because of the way my partner treats me."

  The goal of the previous two chapters has been to help you become clearer as to whether you are being emotionally abused and to help you identify the types of abuse you have been experiencing. It is particularly beneficial to know exactly which tactics your partner uses in order to keep you confused, off-balance, and feeling bad about yourself. When you can begin to recognize your partner's behavior as being abusive, you will be less inclined to believe his words and be manipulated by him. The next two chapters will help you better understand the role of shame in emotional abuse and will undoubtedly help you understand yourself and your reactions and behavior better.

CHAPTER 4

How Shaming Works as a Means of Gaining Control

Shame is a soul-eating emotion.

—CARL JUNG

SOME OF YOU FEEL A great deal of shame because your partner is unhappy with you, and, quite frankly, you don't blame him or her. You feel like a failure as a partner, spouse, and/or parent, even though you are constantly trying to improve. Others are aware of feeling shame as a result of your partner's treatment of you. You recognize that he or she is being emotionally abusive, and you understand that a great deal of his emotionally abusive behavior involves shaming you.

Many of you are quite familiar with the feeling of shame. You've felt it all your life. Others aren't clear about what shame is or how it feels. Whatever your situation, in this chapter, and throughout the rest of the book, we will work toward removing the shame that victims of emotional abuse tend to experience, whether it is the shame that comes from being abused or the shame you brought into the relationship.

As we move forward, I will go into more detail about the emotion of shame, how it creates the primary damage associated with emotional abuse, and how it is often the main reason someone becomes abusive. What most people don't understand is that abuse—any kind of abuse—originates with shame. For years now, those in the therapeutic and recovery communities have identified abuse as being about power and control, and to a great extent this is absolutely true. But what has been ignored is that *at the core of this need to have power and control is the emotion of shame.*

In addition to shame being the prime motivator of abusers, there is the shame that emotional abuse creates in its victims. Victims of the abuse experience horrendous shame as a result of being constantly criticized, humiliated, ridiculed, belittled, and demeaned. This shame erodes their self-esteem, self-confidence, and sense of self-worth to such an extent that they come to believe they are inadequate, unworthy, and so unlovable that no one else would ever want them. All this creates even more shame and can cause victims to lose any strength or motivation to leave.

Shaming someone can be likened to disarming them, stripping them of their self-esteem, their dignity, and their very humanity. Shaming a partner is the perfect way to gain power and control, and yet it has not been addressed as a specific form of abuse, nor has the specific damage caused by shaming been focused on. More important, healing from this shaming has certainly not been addressed.

In this chapter, I identify shaming as a form of emotional abuse, describe its specific effects, and help you begin to heal from your shame in order to regain your self-confidence, improve your self-image, and become empowered enough to end an abusive relationship. Equally important, I will also focus on helping you to stop shaming yourself if you are not ready to leave your relationship even though you realize you are being poorly treated by your partner.

Shame can make you feel that you are a horrible person—damaged, worthless, and disgusting. It also makes you feel that you are flawed and therefore unworthy of love and acceptance. It makes you turn on yourself. Once you have been adequately shamed by an abusive partner, you feel so bad about yourself that you no longer have the wherewithal to fight back, to take care of yourself, or to end the relationship. At this point, the abuser does indeed have total control.

The reason why shaming someone works so well is because we are wired to connect to and seek acceptance from others—to belong. Shame effectively withdraws that acceptance and connection. Shaming someone, in whatever form it takes, is a way to control the other person by using his or her deeply ingrained need for connection with others to threaten that person with disconnection and rejection.

Shame is at the core of not only the abuse of others but of all violence, whether personal or global. It is shame that motivates people to try to gain power and control over others in the first place. Shaming others is a way for people to compensate for the fact that they feel "less than," most likely because someone else shamed them—robbed them of their dignity and honor. We tend to pass the shame we feel onto others. Shaming someone else make us feel superior to that other person. That is why I believe many have missed the boat by focusing on power and control as the primary motivator of abusive behavior. We need to look underneath this need for power and control to discover its origin—shame.

I call emotional abuse a "prison of shame" because that perfectly describes what occurs in an emotionally abusive relationship. The shaming that an emotional abuser doles out on a constant basis literally creates a prison for the victim. She eventually becomes so weakened by the constant onslaughts that she cannot maintain her equilibrium, is too confused to fight back, and eventually gives up. She surrenders to her abuser's wishes, accusations, and beliefs and becomes his prisoner. If this isn't bad enough, she becomes a prisoner of shame as it slowly eats away at any good feelings about herself that she possesses. She begins to hate herself for not standing up to her abuser and for not leaving. She feels more and more incompetent, and this serves to prove the abuser right. Add to this the shame she feels because she doesn't have the strength to leave and you have a person who has become a prisoner of shame. She feels punished, confined, and trapped.

The Types of Shame

Shame is the most damaging and insidious form of emotional abuse. There are many types of shame that eventually create a prison for victims, including:

- The *immediate shame* that comes from being verbally abused, constantly criticized, demeaned, belittled, or made fun of—especially if it is done in front of other people. The victim feels humiliated and diminished and is ashamed to be seen in such a negative way, especially when the criticism is from someone he loves and trusts.
- The shame that occurs when the victim comes to believe she has *failed to please her partner* and experiences herself as a failure to measure up to what she considers reasonable expectations.
- The shame one feels when *he cannot stand up for himself*. Even if a victim disagrees with his abuser's evaluation of him or he feels that she misunderstands him, he may believe, from earlier experiences—either with his partner or with his family of origin—that it will do no good to speak up.
- The *cumulative shame* that comes from the drip, drip, drip of verbal abuse, criticism, unreasonable expectations, or gaslighting.
- The shame that comes when a victim realizes she has *tolerated unacceptable treatment* for far too long.
- The shame that comes from *keeping the secret of the abuse from family and friends*.

- The shame that the victim feels due to the *judgments of others*—either the judgment that he shouldn't put up with abusive behavior or that he should endure the abuse in order to keep the family together.
- The shame the victim feels if she *goes against her religious or cultural beliefs* by leaving an abusive partner. If she was taught that she should be subservient to men and that she should keep the family together at all costs, she may feel she has betrayed her beliefs. Other religious edicts such as to forgive and forget, to focus on your own sins and let your partner focus on his, and that it is blessed to suffer like Jesus can cause a victim to feel tremendous shame if she ends the abusive relationship. In addition, many who have ended an abusive relationship are shamed, blamed, and even turned away from their church or community.

It Is Shame That Motivates Abusers

As a victim of emotional abuse, you need to primarily focus on your own issues and healing, but it is helpful to understand the dynamics of an abuser so you will stop blaming yourself for the abuse. For this reason, I will offer information later in chapter 9 to help you identify what type of abuser you are dealing with, as well as specific strategies to help you cope with and eventually free yourself from each type of abuser.

While their tactics and even their motives may be different, all emotional abusers have one thing in common: *they are all filled with shame themselves*, often because they were horribly shamed in childhood. We tend to treat people the way we were treated, and this couldn't be truer than it is for most abusers. They tend to treat their partners the way their parents treated them or the way they saw their parents interacting with each other. Some abusers take on the controlling, abusive, shaming ways of one of their parents, believing that this is the way they should act. Others do it less consciously, often not even being aware that they are repeating a parent's abusive behavior.

Many project this shame onto others, especially their partners. For some, the reasoning (although unconscious) goes like this: "If I can shame others first, they won't have a chance to shame me." Others have been so shamed that they build up a defensive wall so no one can reach them. In this way, they actually become shameless: their behavior is no longer dictated by society's rules. They are free to do whatever they want—including abusing and attacking others.

This insidious cycle just creates more victims of abuse. As I stated earlier, shame is a natural reaction to being abused. In fact, abuse, by its very nature, is humiliating and dehumanizing. It is extremely difficult to hear from your partner that he experiences you as being stupid, inadequate, uncaring, selfish, lazy, or any other insult he throws at you without eventually beginning to believe him and feeling ashamed of yourself. Once you are filled with shame, you are much easier to manipulate and control.

Furthermore, when you are being insulted, criticized, controlled, or blamed and you cannot find a way to stand up for yourself, state your case, or make the other person see the reality of the situation, you begin to feel *helpless*. There is a sense of indignity about feeling helpless and an even further sense of humiliation to be seen as helpless in the eyes of another person. You can begin to feel like a helpless animal being held down by a much bigger one. As much as you try to wriggle away, you can't.

As human beings, we want to believe that we have control over what happens to us. When that sense of personal power is challenged by victimization of any kind, we feel humiliated. We believe we should have been able to defend ourselves, and because we weren't able to do so, we feel powerless. This powerlessness causes us to feel humiliated—which leads to shame. This tendency for victims to feel ashamed about their own victimization does the abuser's work for him.

How to Identify Shame

Even though shame is one of the most powerful emotions we can feel, it can be a difficult emotion to identify. While shame can cause you to become angry or sad or afraid, it is actually a stand-alone emotion and is more insidious and more all-encompassing than other emotions. It can take over your entire body and mind. When you feel shame, it is like someone pricked you with a pin and took out all the air in you. You feel deflated and small.

Whether we are consciously aware of it or not, shame is a feeling deep within us of being exposed and unworthy. When we feel shamed, we want to hide. We hang our heads, hunch our shoulders, and curve inward as if trying to make ourselves invisible. Many describe shame as a feeling of wanting to disappear or melt away like the wicked witch in the *Wizard of Oz*. Others describe shame as feeling like they have an anchor pulling them down. They feel heavy, inside and out.

Most people who have been deeply shamed take on the underlying and pervasive belief that they are defective or unacceptable. They feel unlovable or bad. Others feel worthless, like they don't deserve anything good.

Shame can also cause us to feel isolated—set apart from the crowd. In primitive cultures, people were banished from the tribe when they broke society's rules. Being shamed feels like being banished—unworthy to be around others. It can make us want to avoid people or avoid situations where there are people gathered.

Physically, we can respond to shame in a variety of ways. Our stomach can become queasy, we can become disoriented or feel dizzy, and we can experience a sinking feeling. Some people even feel like they have suddenly come down with a fever—thus, the saying "red hot shame."

In addition to feeling shame in the moment, many people store shame in their body. Some feel pain in their heart, others experience a burning feeling in their stomach, and some just feel numb. See if you can locate where you experience and hold shame in your body. It might be a feeling, or you may imagine it as a shape or color.

Here are a few examples of what clients have shared with me:

- "I hold my shame in my posture. I'm always slouching, as if I'm ashamed of myself."
- "I see my shame as this large dark mass, almost taking up my entire insides."
- "I see my shame as a black spot on my heart."
- "It took me quite a while to find shame in my body. That is because it was hiding in a corner where no one could find it. I saw it as a wounded child huddled up, arms over her head to protect herself. That is exactly how I feel when my husband starts in on me."

Healthy Shame Versus Debilitating Shame

Shame is not always damaging. There is healthy shame and then there is debilitating shame. The function of healthy shame is to prevent us from harming our social relationships or to motivate us to repair them. It makes us care what others think of us and helps us determine the social cost of a particular behavior or action.

While everyone experiences shame from time to time and many have issues related to shame, victims of any form of abuse tend to suffer from *debilitating* shame. Debilitating or toxic shame is a type of shame that is so all-consuming that it negatively affects every aspect of people's lives—their perception of themselves, their relationships with others, their ability to be intimate with a romantic partner, their ability to risk and achieve success in their career, and their overall physical and emotional health. Debilitating shame is an irrational feeling of worthlessness, humiliation, and self-loathing that has been inflicted onto someone through repeated traumatic experiences. These traumatic experiences are often rooted in childhood, but they can also be caused by continual emotional abuse.

This type of shame is often referred to as toxic because it permeates and corrupts every level of the human system and has a corrosive effect on the individual's psychological outlook, emotional states, and ability to maintain a positive self-image.

Not only is emotional abuse a particularly potent form of abuse but the debilitating shame that results from it is the most destructive of human emotions. This is why it is so important to work on not only escaping the abuse but also healing the shame that goes hand in hand with it.

Shame is the source of cruelty, violence, and destructive relationships. It is also at the core of many addictions, especially alcohol and drug abuse, sexual addictions, and compulsive overeating, as many victims of emotional abuse turn to alcohol, drugs, or other addictions in order to cope with the abuse.

My client Stephanie turned to food for comfort and escape. "I gained one hundred pounds after I got married. I was so ashamed. My kids were embarrassed to be seen with me, and my husband told me that he was no longer physically attracted to me. I knew I needed to lose weight, but I just couldn't seem to stop eating!"

Stephanie soon came to realize that she used food to push down the shame she felt about being emotionally abused. "The key was that I ate until I no longer felt anything. That's how I dealt with the fact that my husband was abusing me. I hated that I was eating so much, but I hated the reality of the situation I was in even more."

Debilitating shame can damage a person's image of herself in ways that no other emotion can, causing a person to feel deeply flawed, inferior, worthless, and unlovable. If someone experiences enough shame, she can become self-loathing to the point that she becomes self-destructive or even suicidal. This is what happened with my client Sheena.

> I believed my husband when he told me that I was a terrible mother and a terrible wife. He constantly pointed out things I left undone or mistakes I made. He told me I was so incompetent that my children didn't respect me. He made me look foolish in my children's eyes by pointing out my mistakes and inadequacies in front of them. He criticized my cooking, my housekeeping, my looks, my choice of TV programs—everything. And I took it all in. I never once questioned his perceptions or his intentions. I didn't see that he was getting pleasure from my suffering.
>
> At night I would cry for hours, and he would just go into the den so it didn't disturb him. I became so despondent that I started collecting pills so I could commit suicide. I saved all kinds of medicine; I didn't care what—my kids' medicine, my husband's prescriptions. I even stole my mother's blood pressure pills. I didn't know what a fatal dose would be; I just believed that if I took enough I could end the pain.
>
> I don't know what stopped me from taking the pills. I guess it was the thought of what it would do to my kids, even though he'd convinced me they didn't love me.

The Effects of Debilitating Shame

Debilitating shame and self-blame can literally make you sick. Research has shown that shame is tied to stress, particularly when people feel they don't have the power, skill, knowledge, or capability to cope with an event. Stress can even impact the immune system. Researchers like clinical psychologist Mary Turner, Ph.D., explain that our culture has developed a procedure for handling guilt. You acknowledge that you did something wrong, you vow not to repeat the behavior, you atone for your actions, and you accept the consequences. Because of this accepted process of expunging guilt, the emotion doesn't trigger stress and therefore isn't likely to affect the immune system.

However, shame—especially debilitating or persistent shame—is another matter. Feeling helplessness and powerlessness produces high levels of stress-related hormones.

When you encounter a perceived threat, your hypothalamus sets off an alarm system in your body. This system prompts your adrenaline glands to release a surge of hormones, including adrenaline and cortisol. Cortisol, the primary stress hormone, alters immune system responses and suppresses the digestive and reproductive systems as well as growth processes. This complex alarm system also communicates with the brain regions that control mood, motivation, and fear.

Typically, once a perceived threat has passed, hormone levels return to normal. But when stressors are always present and you constantly feel under attack, as in the case of emotional abuse and the shame it causes, the fight-or-flight reaction stays turned on. The long-term activation of the stress-response system and the overexposure to cortisol and other stress hormones can disrupt almost all of the body's processes. This can put you at increased risk of many health problems, including anxiety, depression, digestive problems, headaches, heart disease, sleep problems, weight gain, and memory and concentration impairment.

Shame also has many damaging effects on a person's psyche. It can have devastating effects on people's self-esteem, self-confidence, body image, sexuality, ability to relate to others, and ability and willingness to take care of themselves or defend themselves. Some of these effects can be considered severe and some moderate, but as you will see, all create a situation where a person is severely damaged.

Severe Effects of Shame

Although there is a great deal of overlap and interconnectedness, the severe damage created by shame usually manifests itself
into seven general categories:

1. **Feelings of self-hatred and self-loathing:** This includes
   feeling disgust with oneself or with one's body and feeling undeserving of any good—including love, affection,
   success, or happiness. This self-hatred can lead to sabotaging behaviors and to the following category—
   self-destructiveness.
2. **Self-destructiveness:** This includes thoughts of self-
   harm or actual self-harm or self-mutilation such as
   cutting, burning, or stabbing. It also includes thoughts of
   suicide or actual suicide attempts. In a general sense, victims are often self-destructive in other ways as well,
   including engaging in dangerous activities such as unpro-
   tected sex, reckless driving, driving while intoxicated or
   under the influence of drugs, extreme sports, associating
   with dangerous people, or engaging in criminal behavior.
3. **Self-neglect:** This includes not providing for oneself the
   basic human needs such as adequate food (starving
   oneself, depriving oneself of proper nutrition), water,
   clothing (not protecting oneself from the elements),
   rest, and sleep. It also includes not taking care of necessary dental and medical needs.
4. **Reenacting childhood abuse:** This includes becoming involved with partners or friends who are replicas of one's
   abusers (sometimes even choosing someone who looks
   like one's abuser) or becoming like one's abusers (taking
   on their mannerisms, speech, and behavior) and then
   passing on the abuse to others, usually romantic partners and children. It also includes developing a pattern

of allowing others to abuse you (emotionally, physically, sexually) or allowing others to take advantage of you.

5. **Addictive behavior:** This includes addictions to alcohol, drugs, sex, pornography, shopping, stealing, gambling, and love addictions (a compulsive, chronic craving for romantic love in an effort to gain a sense of security and worth from another person).

6. **Rage:** This is often exhibited as being easily angered, yelling, frequent fighting (both physical and verbal), abuse of children or partners, and road rage. Rage projected outwardly manifests as bitterness and hostility toward others. If rage is held in and directed at oneself, it can lead to depression, self-hatred, self-harm, and self-punishment (see item 1 above).

7. **Isolation:** The shame experienced by victims of emotional abuse can cause them to remain isolated from others. The unconscious or even conscious rational is "If I'm not around other people, I don't risk being further shamed." Isolating behaviors include feeling extremely anxious when it comes to socializing with others, being unable or unwilling to socialize with others, remaining closed up in one's home and seldom going out, and/or remaining withdrawn and therefore being unable to strike up conversations or being unable to respond to overtures from others when out in social situations.

Moderate Effects of Shame

Although the moderate effects of shame do not generally bring as much devastation into the lives of victims of emotional abuse, I don't wish to minimize how painful and life-changing they can be. These common behavior patterns can be quite troublesome and can affect victims' lives in the following significant ways:

- Sensitivity to correction or criticism, easily shamed
- Defensiveness—creating a wall between yourself and others, blocking out criticism
- Tendency to be self-critical, harsh with oneself, unforgiving of oneself
- Perfectionism—again, an attempt to avoid further shaming
- People-pleasing behavior in an attempt to avoid further shaming or abuse
- An inability to speak up for oneself, to say what one really means out of fear of offending or hurting someone and thus risking further shaming.
- Driven to be successful and/or powerful, attempting to gain control over others.
- Lack of motivation (unable to follow through on set goals, plans), confusion (unable to discover what career path to follow, unable to commit to a partner)
- Unreasonably high expectations of self and others.

Now that you understand more about how shame can affect victims of emotional abuse in general, it is important to take the time to consider the various ways it has affected you. You've probably recognized your own behavior and ways of thinking as you've read this chapter, but please take the time to complete the following exercise:

How Has Debilitating Shame Affected You?

- Look over the lists of the severe and moderate effects of shame above and notice which items apply to you. Put a check mark next to each of these items.
- Pay attention to how you feel as you do this assessment. Some of you may already be aware of the ways

shame has affected you, and so this might feel like a validating experience for you (in that it feels good to have someone confirm what you already know to be true). Many of you, however, may not have realized that it was the emotion of shame that caused you to experience these feelings and behaviors. It can feel liberating to finally make sense of what in the past seemed to you (and others) to be unexplainable behavior. It can also feel good to realize that you are not alone—that other victims of emotional abuse experience the same feelings. On the other hand, it can bring up feelings of sadness and anger when you come to realize, in this concrete way, to what extent the abuse and the accompanying shame has affected your life.

Understanding the various ways that shame may have affected you is another giant step toward your healing. Once you can begin to recognize how shame has negatively affected you, you are on your way toward ending the emotional abuse, one way or the other. And knowing that it was inevitable that you would be affected in these ways by the emotional abuse can help you begin to forgive yourself for some of your behaviors and for being unable to end the relationship.

PART II

BREAKING OUT OF YOUR PRISON OF SHAME

CHAPTER 5

Taking Shame Out of the Situation

Don't judge yourself by what others did to you.
—C. KENNEDY, *Omorphi*

IF YOU ARE LIKE MANY victims of emotional abuse, you feel horrendous shame for getting into an emotionally abusive relationship in the first place and even worse shame because you are unable to end the relationship. Not only do you suffer from self-induced shame, but you also are likely often shamed by others with questions and comments like "Why do you stay?" or "I would never stay with someone who treats me like your husband treats you."

Those women who have careers and have the financial resources to leave feel particularly shamed by their situation. As one client shared with me: "I'm a success in my career. Other women look to me for advice. I could leave my husband at any time; I'm not trapped like a lot of women are by a lack of money. So I feel a lot of shame when I realize I'm staying in a relationship that is so destructive to me."

Men who are being emotionally abused are in the unique situation of realizing that others expect them to be tough and strong and to never put up with abusive behavior from their wives or girlfriends. One of my male clients told me, "I can't tell anyone about my situation because they will either laugh at me or call me a weakling. People just don't understand it when it is a man who is being abused by his wife. They just think, 'What's wrong with him? Why doesn't he just leave?'"

For the above reasons and because shame can be so debilitating, I have devoted this entire chapter to helping you stop blaming and shaming yourself for choosing an emotionally abusive partner and for your inability to leave.

There should be absolutely no shame in the fact that you are in an emotionally abusive relationship. Victims of emotional abuse cover a wide range of ages, races, social status, economic status, genders, and sexual preferences. *Anyone can be emotionally abused.* It doesn't matter how smart you are, how powerful you are, or how much money you have. You can still be vulnerable to becoming involved with an emotional abuser.

You were not stupid or naïve for becoming attracted to an abusive person. Many smart, well-educated, and savvy women and men have found themselves in your situation. Most abusers present themselves as caring, emotionally healthy individuals, not the shame-inducing, controlling, and manipulating people that they turn out to be. So stop blaming yourself for not seeing through their facade or for not recognizing the abusive side to your partner.

Vulnerable People as Targets

Women and men who are especially vulnerable due to illness, the loss of a loved one, or a recent trauma are often the target of an emotionally abusive person. My client Alma experienced terrible shame because she married a man who almost destroyed her emotionally.

> Five years ago, I was raped and brutally beaten by a stranger. I was left for dead in an alleyway, but fortunately a kind stranger found me and called an

ambulance. That was the day I met my husband. He was the doctor who attended to me at the hospital where I was admitted. He was so loving and so caring toward me. After what I just went through, you'd think I would be afraid of any man who came near me, and basically I was. But this doctor was so quietly attentive that he disarmed me. I ended up trusting him in a way I had never trusted anyone in a long time.

After I left the hospital, the doctor continued to contact me just to ask how I was doing. He brought me food and sat with me when I cried. I'd never been treated so tenderly, and I found myself falling in love with him.

Unfortunately, Alma's husband turned out to be one of the worst type of abusers—the kind who deliberately preys on vulnerable people. During the four years that she was married to him, Alma's husband emotionally tortured her to the point that she almost had to be hospitalized for psychiatric problems.

He made me a prisoner in my own home. I couldn't go out of the house without him. He locked me in the closet if I questioned him. He liked to have total control over me, and he loved seeing me be helpless and powerless. He forced me to have sex with him, sometimes tying my hands behind my back and torturing me with hot wax. He was pure evil. I didn't think I was going to escape from him alive.

Alma's story is extreme, but it is not unusual in the sense that many emotionally abusive partners set out to find vulnerable people they can control and abuse. These abusers present themselves as caring human beings in public—fine, upstanding people in the community and people in power positions like Alma's husband, people you would never imagine could be as abusive as they are.

Betrayal Trauma

Still another reason why emotional abusers can be difficult to spot is the fact that many victims of emotional abuse experienced what is referred to as "betrayal trauma" as a child or adolescent. Betrayal trauma happens when someone whom you trust and who should be trustworthy betrays you, for example, sexual abuse by parents and other caretakers. These early experiences of personal violation interfere with a victim's developing social capabilities, most specifically the ability to make healthy decisions about whom to trust. This puts them at an increased risk of making inaccurate trust decisions in interpersonal relationships, elevating their risk of revictimization. Betrayal trauma results in damaged trust mechanisms, which are linked to a decreased capacity to feel the anticipatory anxiety that usually accompanies dangerous situations. In other words, those who have experienced betrayal trauma experience an inability to decipher potentially emotionally unhealthy situations. In addition, someone with trust deficits can experience the following:

· A limited ability to engage in proper self-defense actions
· A limited ability to self-protect
· An inability to end a physically or emotionally abusive relationship

Other Reasons Why You Were Attracted to an Abusive Partner

There are many other good reasons why you were attracted to an abusive person and why you didn't recognize signs of abusive behavior, including:

- It is quite common for people to become involved with emotional abusers without realizing it because the abuser's controlling and shaming tactics are often subtle and not easily recognized.
- Abusers often appear to be caring and loving at first. In fact, some of them truly are. But gradually, using a wide range of strategies, they become more and more controlling and shaming.
- As it was with Alma's husband, some types of abusers actually have a hidden dark side that they deliberately keep from most people. It isn't until they become emotionally and intimately involved with someone that this side of them comes out. Otherwise, the average person would describe them as kind and caring.
- Unlike some of your previous boyfriends or girlfriends who were unwilling to commit, your abusive partner may have seemed to be open to a committed relationship right away; that is, he or she may have wanted to be with you almost all the time. This can be very attractive, especially if you've had a history of being neglected by your parents or being involved with people who would not commit.
- Your partner may have initially put you on a pedestal, telling you over and over how wonderful you are and how he had never met anyone like you. This is especially inviting to those with low self-esteem or a history of being criticized by parents or previous partners.
- Most people tend to get married or to begin a long-term committed relationship because they have the experience of feeling unconditionally accepted by their partner, some people perhaps for the first time in their life. If you didn't feel loved unconditionally as a child, the experience of having someone love you and accept you unconditionally as an adult is particularly powerful and

can leave you feeling very vulnerable. And many emotional abusers can be extremely manipulating and adept at using a person's vulnerability against them.

Lovebombing

These last three items on the above list fall under the category of what has been called *lovebombing*. This is a deliberate tactic of some abusers to disarm an individual's natural guardedness toward strangers. The abuser creates an intense atmosphere of affection and adoration in order to accelerate feelings of intimacy in the targeted person instead of allowing feelings to gradually grow. This tactic may include:

- **Flattery, including multiple compliments:** When the victim constantly hears how beautiful, wonderful, and irresistible she is, her ego gets a boost and this actually causes physical and chemical changes to her brain, which serve to cement her attraction to the abuser. Quite often the victim will be someone who suffers from low self-esteem, so this ego boost will be particularly exciting.
- **Dependency:** The abuser will insist on seeing the victim often, taking up more and more of his time and energy and preventing him from seeing other people as often. As contact with others diminishes, the only source of warmth and love available to the victim seems to be his newly found partner. The longer this continues, the deeper under the spell he falls, eventually coming to see the abuser as someone he is unable to live without.
- **Destiny:** The abuser tries to convince the victim that they have something special together. He does this with phrases such as "I've never felt this way about anyone before" and "I think you are my soul mate."

Making Up for All the Pain of Childhood

In addition to the above reasons, many people make the mistake of thinking that their partner is going to make up for all the pain and deficits they suffered as a child, and this can set both abuser and abused up for disappointment and abuse. This need and this expectation are not necessarily conscious, but they can be powerful nonetheless.

My client Carmen's father deserted the family when she was only two years old, and she never saw him again. Carmen always yearned for the father she never knew and felt like there was an empty place in her heart for him. At eighteen, she met Laurence and fell in love with him almost instantly. He was big and strong, and he had an air about him that she found attractive. "I felt safe with Laurence. I knew he would always look out for me, protect me." They got married within months of meeting.

But it wasn't long after they got married that Carmen noticed that not only was Laurence protective of her, but he was possessive as well. Whenever they went out, he always accused her of flirting with other men, and he never wanted her to go out alone. "At first I thought he was being protective, but gradually I began to realize that he didn't trust me. He thought that if I went out alone or with my friends I was going to be talking to guys."

Ever so slowly, Carmen became isolated from her friends and even her family. "For some reason, Laurence didn't like my sister, and he discouraged me from going to see her. I realize now it was because she could see through him."

This all continued for several years. The breaking point for Carmen was when she got pregnant and Laurence started controlling her even more. "I couldn't go anywhere without him or even look at another man. He started calling me a whore and telling me I was going to be a terrible mother. This actually got me to thinking, 'Is he going to be a good father, or will he treat our children the same way he does me?'"

This kind of questioning was the beginning of some real soul-searching for Carmen. In fact, it is what brought her into therapy. We explored her reasons for choosing Laurence, and she was able to realize that it was because she was looking for the father she never had.

"I missed having a father so much. When I met Laurence, he checked all the boxes. He was big and strong, and I felt small next to him and I liked that. He seemed very confident, and I liked his 'take-charge' attitude. Unfortunately, I confused his bravado for confidence, when it really just covered up his insecurities. And his take-charge attitude turned out to be his way of being controlling."

As it was with Carmen, little by little, your partner may have become more critical of you—criticizing everything, including the way you dress, the way you speak, and the way you act around other people. He may have couched his criticism in the form of guidance or teaching or simply as his desire to help you.

Why Didn't I Walk Away?

Just as you should not blame yourself for choosing an abusive partner, you also should not blame yourself for not walking away at the first signs of abuse. After all, you loved your partner and you wanted to give him the benefit of the doubt. You wanted to believe his promises to never treat you like that again. And if you have a history of being blamed and shamed as a child, it was not hard to believe your partner when he told you that you caused him to act this way or that he never acted that way in any of his previous relationships.

Victims of emotional abuse tend to minimize their partner's abusive behavior and the effect it is having on them. For example, despite the fact that your partner's abusive behavior was escalating, you may have assured yourself that *it wasn't that bad*. You may have heard or read stories about intimate partner abuse or domestic violence, horrific stories where the abused partner was battered, tortured, or even murdered, and this may have made it harder for you to recognize that you were being abused as well. After all, your partner never hit you, never pushed you into a wall, never locked you in a room.

Why You Didn't Stand Up for Yourself

Victims of emotional abuse are often criticized for not standing up for themselves when their partner first became abusive. But here too, most abusers are very adept at handling concerns voiced by their partners. Each time you noticed something you didn't like about your partner, he may have passed it off as you being too critical or "making something out of nothing." He may have even listened to your concerns and apologized profusely in order to rein you back in. For example, he apologized for being so jealous and promised to never let it happen again, or he may have explained that he was under a lot of pressure at work and apologized for taking it out on you.

Even as you began to recognize that the troubling behavior was not going away or that it was even getting worse, your partner may have been able to convince you that the problems you were having in the relationship were "normal" and that the two of you just needed to work together to create a better relationship. This usually involved you needing to change in some way in order for him to stop misbehaving. You may have begun to hear the all-too-often-used phrase *"If only you'd do this, I wouldn't do that."*

Eventually, you may have come to realize that the problems were not normal and that, in fact, it wasn't you who needed to change. You may have tried again to bring up his unacceptable behavior. Unfortunately, even this direct approach didn't work. First of all, emotional abusers are often experts at twisting your words and talking circles around you. For example, abusive partners often resort to yelling, cursing, and name-calling when you attempt to stand up to them or push back on their demands. You may have come to the conclusion that if you want to keep the peace it is better to just comply with your partner's wishes.

Still another tactic an abusive partner uses when confronted is to stomp out of the room and refuse to listen to you. Instead of hearing you out and giving you feedback, she marches out of the room and refuses to talk. Rather than dealing with the issue at hand, abusive partners tend to make a dramatic exit to show you who is boss and to end an uncomfortable discussion.

Another tactic is to use shaming or guilt trips to manipulate you. When victims attempt to stand up to their partners or call them on their offensive behavior, abusers often play the victim and say things to you like: "I can't believe you really believe this about me. Don't you know that all I want is to make you happy? But no matter what I do, you are never satisfied. Frankly, I wonder if you are incapable of being happy."

Let's say that you have grown increasingly uncomfortable with the fact that your partner repeatedly puts you down in front of others. You approach him after a recent incident and ask him to stop doing this. Instead of talking about it with you, instead of admitting that he did this, instead of apologizing and promising to work on not doing it again, he is likely to deny it profusely, act like he is hurt at the accusation, or stomp off, showing you that your complaint is not worth a serious, mature conversation.

Reasons Why It Is Difficult to End an Emotionally Abusive Relationship

It can feel even worse once you have become certain that you are being emotionally abused and that you are being damaged by the experience. Many of my clients, after realizing they are indeed being emotionally abused, feel horrible shame because they aren't able to leave.

"I wish I wasn't so clear about the fact that I am being abused," one client told me. "At least I could pretend it wasn't happening before. But now I know I need to end the relationship, and I feel so ashamed that I can't do it."

There is no shame in the fact that you are having a difficult time ending the relationship. You love him, and you've built a life together. And you may doubt whether you can make it on your own, both financially and emotionally. You probably have a lot less confidence than you had when you met your partner. You've been beaten down and manipulated to the point that you don't trust yourself to be able to take care of yourself and/or your children.

Still another reason why many victims have a difficult time leaving is that they are overwhelmed with confusion. Cynthia started therapy because she was confused about whether or not she should leave her husband. They had been married for two years, and she explained that he was a real Dr. Jekyll and Mr. Hyde.

"Before we married, James was the most loving, considerate man you'd ever want to meet. But now he is impatient and critical. He complains about everything—the way I dress, the way I cook, the way I clean the house. He seems to look for things to criticize. The other day he got on me because he found something old in the back of the refrigerator! Before we were married, we used to have long conversations, but now when I offer my opinion about something, he treats me like I'm a child or like I'm stupid and just dismisses what I say."

Cynthia explained that if her husband acted in these ways all the time she would know for certain that she should divorce him. But he keeps her off balance by sometimes reverting back to the way he was before they got married. "It is so confusing. Sometimes he can still be so sweet to me. He tells me he loves me, and he says he's sorry for being so critical of me. His father was critical of him, and he knows how much it hurts. He's been there for me with some problems I've had with my parents, and he's been really good to my daughter, who lives with us."

It took some time for Cynthia to come to the conclusion that her husband was emotionally abusing her. She also needed to understand that the longer she stayed with her husband, the worse she was going to feel about herself and the more confused and disoriented she would become. But even when she was able to face these things, she still couldn't leave.

Common reasons why victims don't end an emotionally abusive relationship include:

- They blame themselves for all the problems in the relationship.
- They come to believe the abuser and are now convinced that they are too stupid, incompetent, ugly, or unlovable for anyone else to ever want them
- They have come to believe they cannot make it on their own.
- The abuser has threatened to tell everyone they abuse their children or to take the kids away from them or even kill them.
- They are afraid to be alone.
- They have a history of being abused or shamed, and so it feels normal to them.

Take a close look at the reasons listed above and see if you relate to one or more of them. If you do, please remind yourself that these are common reasons why victims of emotional abuse stay and that they are, in fact, good reasons.

A History of Abuse or Shaming

The last item on the above list is particularly important and can be one of the main reasons why you have stayed in an abusive relationship. Many people have suffered from a heavy dose of shame before they enter an emotionally abusive relationship as an adult. Because of this, shaming may feel normal to you. For many, the root of this shame is abuse. Shame and the damage it does to childhood victims is the primary reason why former victims of child abuse or neglect may stay in emotionally abusive relationships as adults.

Unfortunately, shaming was an integral part of many people's upbringing since many parents (and other caretakers) believe that shaming a child is an acceptable and even beneficial form of discipline.

There are many ways that parents shame their children. These include:

BELITTLING: Comments from parents like "You're such a crybaby" or "I'm ashamed to be seen with you" are horribly humiliating to a child. It is also humiliating when a parent makes a negative comparison between her child and another child, such as "Why can't you act like Bobby? He isn't a crybaby." This is not only humiliating, but it also teaches a child to always compare himself with peers and find himself deficient in the comparison.

BLAMING: When a child makes a mistake, it is important for her to take responsibility for her action. But many parents go way beyond teaching the child a lesson by blaming and berating her, telling her "You stupid idiot! You should have known better than to . . ." All this accomplishes is to shame the child to such an extent that she cannot find a way to walk away from the situation with her head held high. Blaming the child like this is like rubbing her nose in the mess she made, and it produces such intolerable shame that she may be forced to deny responsibility or find ways of excusing it.

CONTEMPT: Expressions of disgust or contempt communicate absolute rejection. The look of contempt (often a sneer or a raised upper lip), especially from someone who is significant to a child, can be a devastating inducer of shame because the child is made to feel disgusting or offensive. When I was a child, my mother had an extremely negative attitude toward me. Much of the time, she either looked at me with the kind of expectant look that said "What are you up to now?" or with a look of disapproval or disgust over what I had already done. These looks were very shaming to me, causing me to feel that there was something terribly wrong with me. As a young woman, I was extremely sensitive to what I imagined other people thought of me. I placed an inordinate amount of attention on how I looked. I tended to go along with whatever a male partner wanted, and I was always devastated each time a man ended the relationship, feeling horribly rejected and assuming it was because he had discovered how inadequate or bad I was.

HUMILIATION: As Gershen Kaufman stated in his book *Shame: The Power of Caring,* "There is no more humiliating experience than to have another person who is clearly the stronger and more powerful take advantage of that power and give us a beating." I can personally attest to this. In addition to shaming me with her contemptuous looks, my mother often punished me by hitting me with the limb off a tree, and she often did this outside, in front of the neighbors. The humiliation I felt was like a deep wound to my soul.

DISABLING EXPECTATIONS: Appropriate parental expectations serve as necessary guides to behavior and are not disabling. Disabling expectations, on the other hand, have to do with pressuring a child to excel or to perform a task, skill, or activity. For example, instead of involving their child in a sport for fun, some parents insist that their children "be the best" in the sport, punishing them or rejecting them when they don't perform up to parental expectations. Parents who have an inordinate need to have their children excel at a particular activity or skill are likely to behave in ways that pressure the children to do more and more, such as yelling at them during games or forcing them to continue taking classes or playing a sport when the children clearly show no interest. According to Kaufman, when children become aware of the real possibility of failing to meet parental expectations, they often experience what Kaufman calls "a binding self-consciousness," which means that the children become painfully aware of themselves and their actions and judge themselves harshly. When something is expected of children in this way, attaining the goal is made harder, if not impossible. The more pressure they feel to achieve, the more self-conscious they become, which in turn takes away their focus and their ability to perform. This leads to self-criticism and self-contempt in addition to whatever disapproval and belittling they are receiving from the parent.

TELLING CHILDREN YOU ARE DISAPPOINTED IN THEM: Yet another way that parents induce shame in their children is by communicating to them that they are a disappointment to the parents. Such messages as "I can't believe you could do such a thing" or "I am deeply disappointed in you," accompanied by a disapproving tone of voice and facial expression, can crush a child's spirit.

HOW WERE YOU SHAMED AS A CHILD?

- Based on the information above, list all the ways your parents or caretakers shamed you as a child.
- Now write more extensively about some of the most shaming experiences you remember. Take your time and remember the incidents or words, providing as much detail as you can. As you write, pay attention to how your body reacts and how you feel emotionally. These feelings and emotions may remind you of how you feel today when your partner uses any of the above tactics to shame you.

- Keep this writing about your childhood shame in a safe place where your partner cannot find it. Better yet, use it to start a journal that you keep under lock and key. This writing will be extremely beneficial as we move along. It will help remind you of how you got where you are today and hopefully help you to stop blaming yourself for not being able to leave.

Other Significant Shaming Experiences

In addition to parental shaming, you may have previously been shamed by any or all of the following:

- Shame from child abuse, neglect, and abandonment
- Shame from previous emotionally or physically abusive relationships as an adult
- Other traumas, such as sexual assault as an adolescent or adult

Childhood Abuse

Research shows that shame is an emotion that is highly characteristic of victims of childhood abuse, who tend to belittle and degrade themselves. Victimized children often believe that they brought the abuse on themselves and that they do not deserve to be loved unconditionally. This belief tends to be carried forward into their adult relationships.

Furthermore, research suggests that adults, particularly women, who were victimized as children are at risk of revictimization in later life. For example, in one famous survey, it was found that 72 percent of women who experienced either physical or sexual abuse as a child also experienced violence in adulthood, compared with 43 percent of women who did not experience child abuse.

In general, those who experienced any form of child abuse or neglect are particularly vulnerable when it comes to being re-victimized. This is true for several important reasons:

- **An impaired sense of self:** Women and men who experienced childhood abuse often have an impaired sense of self. This can cause you to look to the reactions of others to gauge how you are feeling about a situation, and because of this you may be gullible and easily manipulated by others. You may be unable to establish appropriate boundaries, even with your own children. In addition, you may have difficulty asking others for help, creating or finding a support network, or taking advantage of support that is available.

- **Avoidance:** Avoidance symptoms can help you cope by temporarily reducing emotional pain. Some of the more serious symptoms related to avoidance are substance abuse, compulsive high-risk sexual activities, eating disorders, and self-injurious behaviors. One of the most common types of avoidance is *dissociation*—a way to "escape" from abuse and pain. Adult survivors often describe being able to numb their bodies or "watch" the abuse from above their body while they are being abused. As a child, this may have been the way you survived sexual or physical abuse—the way you emotionally coped with unbearable physical and/or emotional pain. But dissociation can become an unconscious habit and can therefore not only remove you from uncomfortable or abusive situations but also add to your tendency to deny that abuse is occurring. If you aren't present in your own body, you will put up with abuse for far too long. While you may not be

consciously aware of the abuse or its consequences, it
doesn't mean you aren't being negatively affected.

- **Cognitive distortion:** Cognitive distortions are ways that
  our mind convinces us of something that isn't true. For
  example, if you suffered abuse or neglect in childhood,
  you may view the world as a dangerous place. Because
  you were powerless in the past, you may underestimate
  your own sense of self-efficacy and self-worth in dealing
  with danger, and therefore *feel that there is nothing you can
  do when faced with difficult situations*. You may feel powerless to protect yourself.
- **Low self-esteem:** Research shows that women in particular who experienced childhood violence or who witnessed
  parental violence could be at risk of being victimized as
  adults as they are more likely to have low self-esteem.
- **Violence is normalized:** Those who grow up in households where one parent emotionally or physically abuses
  the other may come away believing that violent behavior
  is a normal response to dealing with conflict.

Neglect

Research shows that childhood neglect increases a person's
vulnerability to intimate partner violence in adulthood. More specifically, adults with documented histories of childhood neglect
were found to have an increased risk for a greater number and variety of acts of psychological abuse from an intimate partner. In
one significant study, it was found that experiencing neglect as a
child interferes with a person's ability to enter into nonabusive intimate partner relationships.

Emotional neglect, in particular, can have a great impact on a
child—surprisingly, as much of an impact as physical or sexual
abuse. Childhood emotional neglect happens when a parent fails

to respond to a child's emotional needs. Even though the parent may take care of the child overall, something invisible is missing: the parent doesn't validate the child's feelings or respond to the child's emotional needs.

Emotionally neglected children can end up feeling deeply alone. As kids, they feel their needs aren't important, that their feelings don't matter, or that they should never ask for help (either because it is perceived as a sign of weakness or because they believe it is hopeless). As they grow up, they tend to experience unnecessary guilt, self-anger, low self-confidence, or a sense of being deeply, personally flawed.

If you were emotionally neglected as a child, think about how that experience could have caused you to be vulnerable to an emotional abuser as an adult, either because he or she seemed to hold the promise of your receiving the love and attention you didn't get from your parents or because you expected so little from a partner given the little you received as a child.

Child Sexual Abuse

While all abuse is shaming, child sexual abuse can be especially shaming. Long-term effects include depression, suicidal tendencies, sexual dysfunction, self-mutilation, chronic anxiety, post-traumatic stress disorder, dissociation, memory impairment, somatization, and impairment in interpersonal functioning. But the most significant consequence of childhood sexual abuse is debilitating shame.

There are many reasons why childhood sexual abuse victims experience a great deal of shame.

- There is the shame that is created any time a person is victimized because the act of victimization causes a person to feel helpless and this helplessness creates a feeling of shame.

- There is the shame that comes when a child's body is invaded in such an intimate way by an adult or older child.
- There is the shame associated with being involved with something that the child knows is taboo or, as many children describe it, doing something that makes them feel "icky."
- There is the shame that comes over a child who is "betrayed" by his or her body when it responds to the touch of the perpetrator.

It is important to acknowledge just how much childhood sexual abuse influences and even forms former victims' personalities, their ability to protect themselves from further sexual and other violations, and even their motivation to do so. Former victims of childhood sexual abuse are often unable to stand up for themselves and adequately protect themselves. This is because the effects of this type of abuse are devastating to a young girl's or boy's self-esteem, self-confidence, and self-concept. Furthermore, the trauma can make it difficult for former victims to believe they deserve to be protected and respected.

Not only does abuse in childhood and childhood sexual abuse in particular create an enormous amount of shame in a person, but having experienced these forms of abuse also can actually set a person up to be re-victimized in adulthood. Numerous studies have reported a relationship between child abuse and neglect and the perpetration of intimate partner violence. In fact, at least one study, the Toledo Adolescent Relationships Study, found that child abuse predicted intimate partner violence.

Furthermore, the emotional experience of shame and the tendency to self-blame have been shown to have a significant relationship to re-victimization in general. The way you explain a negative event to yourself—the explanation you have as to why a bad thing happened to you—can strongly influence how you feel about yourself, making you feel like a bad person who deserved the abuse or that you actually caused it.

Many of you reading this book have clear memories of being abused or neglected as a child. But some people's memories are not so clear, and some people question the memories they do have. Many have not labeled their experiences as abuse or neglect, even though it is clearly what they experienced. If you are uncertain whether you were abused or neglected as a child or are not sure what constitutes abuse, I suggest you check out the complete list offered in my book *It Wasn't Your Fault: Freeing Yourself from the Shame of Childhood Abuse with the Power of Self-Compassion.*

Your Shame Story

- Make a list of all the shaming and abuse experiences you can remember from your childhood and your adulthood so far. It can be an extremely powerful experience to view all your shaming experiences in black and white. Note: Don't expect yourself to create this list in one sitting. It may take days or even weeks to complete it. In fact, it isn't healthy or constructive to make this list all at once.
- Using this list, write your "Shame Story." Describe how each of these shaming events felt and how you believe you have been affected by each one. Again, don't write your entire shame story in one sitting. Write about one experience or one time in your life and allow yourself to digest it and feel any emotions attached to it before attempting to write about another experience. You don't want to overwhelm yourself with your feelings by trying to do it all at one time.

· After you have completed your shame story, read it out loud to yourself. As you do so, pay attention to what emotions you feel and what is happening in your body. Your shame story can be a powerful reminder of what you have been through in your life, the suffering you have endured. Allow yourself to feel whatever emotions bubble up. We will be discussing the importance of self-compassion in later chapters, but for now begin to offer yourself healing compassion for your pain. You can do this by simply saying to yourself:

It is so sad that I suffered from so much shame as a child.

or

No wonder I got involved with an emotionally abusive partner; I was repeating what was done to me in childhood.

Processes like this exercise will help you gain a deeper understanding of yourself and your behavior. It will also help you gain compassion for your suffering, not just for what you have experienced from your current partner but also for what you likely endured as a child. We will discuss more about the benefits of such self-compassion in chapter 8, but for now, know that the more you understand yourself, the more you can heal your shame from the past and present.

ALL THE CAUSES described in this chapter are valid explanations as to why you chose your partner and why you are still in an abusive relationship. Please write down all the causes mentioned in this chapter that apply to you. Then the next time you begin to chastise yourself for remaining in an emotionally abusive relationship, you can remind yourself of these valid and compelling reasons.

In response to your own self-criticism or the criticism of others as to why you don't leave, begin to tell yourself the following:

It is understandable *that I would
have chosen someone like my partner.*
or
It is understandable *that I am unable
to leave my partner at this time.*

Please note: even though I have outlined many of the reasons why you may have unconsciously chosen an abusive partner and why you may find it so hard to end the relationship based on childhood neglect or abuse, this does not mean the abuse is your fault. And some people are emotionally abused even when they weren't abused or neglected in childhood.

CHAPTER 6

Stop Believing the Abuser

*But better to get hurt by the truth than comforted with
a lie.*

—KH KHALED HOSSEINI, *The Kite Runner*

MANY OF MY CLIENTS WERE originally unaware of the fact that
they were being emotionally abused. In fact, most who come
into counseling want me to fix them so they will be a better partner or parent. They often ask "What's wrong with me?" "Why
can't I do what my husband asks me to do?" "Why can't I prove
to my wife that I love her?" and "Why can't I do things right?"

What becomes abundantly clear once clients begin to describe
their life with their partner is that the problem is not that they are
too lazy or too selfish or that they don't want to have sex enough
with their partner or any of the other complaints their partner has
about them; the problem usually lies in the *unreasonable expectations* of their partner or in the *distorted way* their partner views
himself or herself, others, and the world.

Those who are being abused tend to believe that when their
partner complains about something, it is because they are, in fact,
doing something wrong. For instance, it doesn't occur to a woman
that her husband or boyfriend is complaining because he has a
need to make her feel bad about herself. She doesn't suspect that
her partner focuses on her real or imagined faults so he won't
have to focus on his own. People don't understand that abusers

blame their partners so they don't have to feel guilty about the things they have done or take responsibility for their own problems, weaknesses, and faults. And it certainly doesn't dawn on victims that their partner may be an entitled narcissist who has to have everything his way and who will never be pleased. Most important, *they don't understand that as long as their partner shames them, he or she doesn't have to feel their own shame.* Neither does it occur to them that their partner may see them through a distorted lens due to the fact that he or she suffers from borderline personality disorder or borderline traits.

Because all the above may be true, it is important that you come to believe and understand the following: *most abusers do not criticize you because they have your best interest at heart, nor do they have the best interest of your relationship at heart.* Abusers are focused on their own self-interest, and unfortunately, they are often focused on making you feel "less than" them. Once you have absorbed this truth, it will be the beginning of you taking on a totally new perspective when it comes to your partner.

Instead of assuming that what your partner says about you is true, question his or her motives. Ask yourself:

- What will my partner gain from convincing me that something is wrong with me?
- How does my partner benefit by blaming me for everything that goes wrong?
- How does it benefit my partner to make me doubt myself?
- What is the benefit in convincing me that I am not good enough?

Your answers to these questions can be very revealing. Coming to realize that your partner's motives are suspect will make it harder for him to control you with his complaints, assessments, and innuendos.

So the first step in being able to inoculate yourself against emotional abuse is to *stop always believing what your partner tells you*. Stop taking your partner's words to heart and stop taking your partner's abusive actions and words personally. Instead, it is important that you come to understand that *your partner's perceptions, evaluations, and beliefs are faulty, distorted, and extremely unreasonable.*

This may seem like a radical stance to take. After all, your partner can't always be wrong. Some of the things she tells you about yourself seem accurate. She seems to know you better than anyone else because she can see through what she calls your manipulations and lies. She knows your history and knows what "you are capable of." And she isn't always critical or unreasonable. Sometimes she is loving and caring, and because of this you believe she really cares about you.

As radical as it may seem to make the blanket statement that *you need to stop believing your partner*, this is what you need to do in order to balance out your tendency to *always believe* her. This is what you need to do to get out from under her control.

If you are like most victims of emotional abuse, you suffer from an excess of accountability: you already believe everything is your fault. This makes you extremely vulnerable to blaming, manipulation, and lies. You don't need your partner reinforcing the idea that you are always wrong. The chances are high that you already believe this. In fact, what you need is the opposite. You need to begin to believe that *you are not always the cause of the problem.* You need to realize that you couldn't possibly be as bad as your partner makes you out to be. No one constantly messes up the way you are being accused of doing it.

It will not be an easy task to move from always believing your partner to recognizing that you cannot necessarily trust his words. It can be difficult to suddenly begin to look at and listen to your partner from this different perspective. This chapter will help you to make this important transition.

The Lies You Are Being Told

When I use the word *lies*, I am referring to more than the act of telling a falsehood. I'm also talking about creating an atmosphere of dishonesty, blaming, faultfinding, projecting, gaslighting, and scapegoating. Lies can take all kinds of forms, including out-and-out falsehoods, exaggerations, distortions, and projections. Here is a list of the most common forms of lying that abusive people engage in:

LIE #1:   "I'm a man, so you need to do as I say."

LIE #2:   "I'm better than you, and therefore I deserve to be treated special."

LIE #3:   "I'm smarter than you, and therefore you should believe everything I say."

LIE #4:   "I need to advise you (or teach you) because you aren't capable of making good decisions on your own."

LIE #5:   "You're too stupid (or crazy) to understand what you are doing. You need me to tell you when you make a mistake; otherwise you'd never realize it."

LIE #6:   "I had a horrible childhood, so you need to make up for what I didn't receive."

LIE #7:   "You don't even recognize how bad you treat me. You need me to spell it out for you."

LIE #8:   "You can't be trusted, so I have to watch you carefully and question your every move."

LIE #9:   "You're not who I thought you were when I married you."

LIE #10:   "You don't meet my needs/expectations, so you need to work on improving yourself."

LIE #11:   "You hurt my feelings (or disappointed me), and now you have to make up for it."

LIE #12:   "It's your responsibility as my wife/girlfriend to satisfy my every sexual need and desire."

Although your partner may not use these exact words, it is the underlying message that is important to note. As you will notice, all of these lies center around four basic ideas: (1) I am superior to you, (2) you are incapable or incompetent, (3) you are untrustworthy, and (4) you owe me.

Of all the ways abusers create an atmosphere of dishonesty, the most common strategies are lying, projecting, and gaslighting. Let's examine each one separately, starting with lying.

Lying

Some abusers actually believe their own lies; others know they are lying but are bent on convincing you that their lies are true. The way the typical abuser views his or her partner and relationship is based on three major lies: (1) You are responsible for your partner's happiness, (2) you are responsible for your partner's anger, and (3) you are responsible for fixing the relationship. Let's examine each of these major lies in more depth.

1. **You are responsible for your partner's happiness:** This lie plays on your natural, healthy desire to please your mate. But it is absolutely not true. No one is responsible for a partner's happiness. You can do all you can to help your partner feel loved and secure, but ultimately it is your partner's responsibility to make himself or herself happy. And unfortunately, abusive people often have *unreasonable expectations* when it comes to what they feel makes them happy.

   Your partner may have the following unreasonable expectations of you:
   - That you focus all your attention on her
   - That you put his needs ahead of your own, or even your children's

· That you view him as your boss and that he has the final word in all decisions.

The bottom line is that no matter how hard you try, there are people who will never be happy, and so your attempts to please them will be for naught. Abusers are often depressed, insecure, inadequate people who have serious mental health issues that you cannot solve.

2. **You are responsible for creating the abuser's anger:** Abusive partners believe that it is your fault whenever they become angry. If only you had done such and such or not done such and such, they wouldn't have gotten angry. And because you made them angry, their emotionally (or physically) abusive behavior is justified. The solution to the problem as far as they are concerned: just don't make them angry. Do whatever they want, don't question them, don't dare to cross them, don't dare to disagree with them. This lie puts the abusive partner in the role of a parent, a boss, or the authority. And it puts the abused partner on the defensive, causing intense self-monitoring, second-guessing, and self-blaming.

3. **You are responsible for fixing the relationship:** Because abusers cannot or will not acknowledge their own problems or issues, they project them onto others, especially their partner. And because, as far as they are concerned, the relationship problems all center around you, you have to be the one to solve them. But the chances are very high that you play no role in your partner's problems and only a small role in the relationship problems. Yes, you've heard many times that relationships are a two-way street and that there are always two sides to a story, and of course, there is truth to these concepts. But the stronger truth is that you don't cause your partner to become abusive. (No one does.) He came into the relationship with issues and problems that caused him to

be abusive. And even though we typically think that it is the responsibility of both partners to fix a broken relationship, the truth is that it is always the abuser's responsibility to stop being abusive. Even though you may have tolerated or enabled his behavior for far too long, you are not responsible for stopping it. He is.

Abusers often use your understanding and/or forgiving nature to manipulate you into believing the lie that you are responsible for fixing the relationship. They often do this by saying some version of the following: "You need to be more understanding because you know I had a rough childhood" or "You need to forgive me." These two phrases, or some version of them, are particularly powerful, causing many partners to put up with behavior no one should ever be subjected to.

Many victims of emotional abuse stay in the relationship because of guilt or obligation despite the damage the relationship has done to their own mental health. This is what my client Marty told me when I asked why he stays with his wife even though he is extremely unhappy.

> My wife had a horrible childhood. She was sexually abused by her stepfather, and when she told her mother, she accused her of lying. So she has a lot of issues, and she can't help the way she acts. For example, she becomes enraged if she ever feels like I'm putting someone else ahead of her or if I ever seem to take someone else's side, even our children's. And she has trust issues; she's extremely jealous and possessive. She often accuses me of flirting with other women or being unfaithful to her and flies into a rage and starts screaming and yelling. I try not to take it personally, but when I don't admit whatever it is that she is accus-

> ing me of, she calls me a liar and gives me the silent
> treatment for days. I have the hardest time with this,
> but I know she can't help it.

While it is true that Marty's wife cannot control her reactions because she is often triggered based on her abusive childhood and it is wonderful that he has so much compassion for her, the truth is that she needs psychological help. Her partner shouldn't have to sacrifice his own happiness (and mental health) in order to support her.

The sad truth is that you may have come into the relationship already believing the three major lies we have discussed. Your partner's beliefs and expectations may have only reinforced your own. You may have put your partner on a pedestal, giving him far more power than he deserves. If he is better educated or more accomplished, you may have assumed he knew more than you on nearly all subjects. And if you were raised in an extremely religious or conservative home where the man of the house had all the power, you may have naturally given this power to your male partner.

Projection

For the most part, your partner knows when she is lying. She does it deliberately to make you feel bad about yourself or doubt yourself, to stay in a one-up position with you, or to cover her tracks when she has done something wrong, such as cheating. But there is a form of lying that abusers engage in that is not necessarily deliberate, and this is *projection*.

Projection is a defense mechanism in which a person protects her ego by denying the existence of a characteristic or feeling within herself by attributing the trait to others. For example, a person who is habitually rude to others accuses other people of being rude, someone who is threatened by her own angry feelings often accuses her partner of harboring hostile thoughts about her. This can be an unconscious defense tactic, meaning she doesn't even realize what she is doing. But the truth is, if people accuse you of being guilty of doing something or acting in a certain way, they don't have to face it in themselves.

Another aspect of this unconscious defense mechanism is that sometimes when a person is aware of doing something wrong, he assumes that others are acting the same way. Therefore, he feels fairly sure of himself when he accuses you of something. For example, it is very common for someone who is cheating on his spouse to accuse his partner of cheating on him.

For years, my client Gina's husband had convinced her that she was so emotionally messed up from her childhood that no one could get along with her. He accused her of being too jealous and possessive and of having serious commitment issues. Gina had extremely low self-esteem and felt insecure, so for years she believed her husband's assessment of her.

When I first began seeing Gina, I asked her if she believed her husband's accusations were always true. She told me that she didn't recognize these behaviors in herself, but that she had never doubted that her husband must be right. "I'm not very self-aware," she told me. "I thought that I must just be so disconnected from myself that I can't see myself clearly."

But as we continued working together, it became abundantly clear that Gina's husband was using *projection* to deflect from the fact that he was actually the one who was jealous and possessive and unable to commit.

As Gina continued in therapy, she began to notice how insecure her husband was. "He hates it that I'm in therapy. He's always nagging at me to quit. I started wondering why he was so set against it, and I began to wonder whether he was afraid I was going to get stronger."

In time, Gina began to notice other things. "I've been feeling better about myself, and so I signed up for a dance class. He didn't like this at all. He insisted on taking me there and picking me up, and I'm sure it was because he was worried I was going to meet someone there. If I talked to a guy after class, he accused me of flirting with him. I began to think that my husband was as insecure as I am. He always accused me of being jealous and possessive, and here he was acting the same way.

"As a way of getting him off my back, I suggested he get involved with an activity so he wouldn't be alone at night. But he said he just wanted it to go back to the way it used to be, both of us spending all our evenings together. I suddenly realized that I wasn't the jealous, insecure one at all. He was. He had convinced me I was these things so he didn't have to deal with his own feelings of insecurity."

Gaslighting

We discussed this phenomenon earlier in the book, in chapter 3, "Tools of the Trade." As noted, this term comes from the film *Gaslight,* in which a husband attempts to drive his wife crazy by making her doubt herself. Gaslighting is an extremely effective form of emotional abuse because it causes victims to question their own feelings, perceptions, memory, instincts, reality, and even their sanity. Being tricked into not trusting yourself may be the biggest lie of all. This gives the abusive partner a lot of power and control. Once an abusive partner has broken down the victim's ability to trust his or her own perceptions, the victim is more likely to put up with abusive behavior and stay in the relationship.

It can be extremely difficult to catch your partner when he is gaslighting you. In fact, that is what gaslighting is designed to do— confuse you. In order to help you cut through the confusion, here are some signs that your partner is gaslighting you.

- He denies he said something you are sure he said: "I didn't say that. You're imagining things."

- She denies she did something you are sure she did: "I didn't spend that money; you must have."
- He denies that something happened: "Are you sure that's what happened? You have a bad memory, you know."
- He accuses you of making too much of something or being too sensitive: "Are you going to get angry over a little thing like that?"
- She turns the tables and accuses you of the behavior she is guilty of: "I don't have an anger problem; you're the one who is always angry with me!"
- He causes you to question your memory by correcting your recollections: "That's not the way it happened. It happened like this."
- He blames you for his mistakes. "The reason I'm late is because you forgot to fill up the gas tank and I had to stop at the gas station."

In order to overcome this form of abuse, you must start recognizing the signs and work on learning to trust yourself again. The signs that you are being a victim of gaslighting include:

- You often feel confused.
- You constantly doubt yourself.
- You question whether what he has accused you of is right.
- You seriously question whether you are going crazy.
- You doubt your own perceptions and reality.
- You question your memory.
- Even though you don't see yourself the way your partner sees you, you wonder whether he is right.
- You have the sense that you used to be a different person—more confident, more relaxed, and fun-loving.

How to Counter These and Other Lies

As difficult as it can be to stop believing your partner's lies, it starts with you no longer believing your partner's put-downs, his so-called suggestions for your own good, and his evaluations of who you are. He may have been slowly manipulating you for months and often years to believe that what he says is the absolute truth—that he sees you better than anyone else ever has. But the real truth is, he is absolutely wrong. He doesn't see you better than anyone else because he sees you through a lens of shame—his own shame. The shame he wants to pass on to you so that he doesn't have to feel it.

Many abusers put themselves out there as experts, teachers, or enlightened ones. Here are some common lies these type of abusers tell their partners:

- "It's for your own good."
- "I know what is best for you. You have terrible judgment."
- "Just do it my way. I know what I'm doing and you don't."
- "I know what I'm talking about; you don't."

Sound familiar? If the abuser focuses on what he thinks is wrong with you enough, he doesn't have to deal with his own problems, he doesn't have to address his own shortcomings. He can remain the expert, the teacher, the enlightened person who is just trying to help you, who is just trying to get you to see the error of your ways so that he can love you. But it is vitally important that you to come to know this truth: *love isn't about trying to make your partner a better person; it is about making yourself a better person.* When we truly love someone, we want to make necessary changes in ourselves so that the relationship works for both people. If your partner is emotionally abusing you, he is certainly not working on improving himself.

How to Stop Believing Your Partner's Put-Downs

In order to stop believing your partner's put-downs, negative assessments, and unwanted advice, you will need to begin to take the following steps.

Stop Giving Your Partner So Much Power over You

There may have always been an imbalance of power in your relationship. It is common for those who are being emotionally abused to be attracted to partners who seem to know more than they do, who seem far more confident and sure of themselves than they feel. In fact, this may have been part of their original appeal. When we don't feel confident and secure, it can feel comforting to be around someone who seems to express these things. It can make us feel safe, protected. If we don't feel intelligent or we are not educated or successful, someone who is all these things can be very attractive, and having them be attracted to you can feel like a compliment. If you have a difficult time socially and find it difficult to converse with others, someone who is charming and who connects with and talks with others easily can be very alluring. You no longer have to feel like the wallflower in the corner. He brings you into the conversation, he lifts you up in front of others. And so from the beginning, you may have given your partner too much power. You may have put him on a pedestal.

However, maybe the power imbalance developed over time. There may have been a gradual shifting of power so that you have ended up feeling "less than" him. He may have become increasingly opinionated and controlling. Maybe once you were married, he insisted that he be the "man of the house" and that you do what he says. You may have quit your job to be a fulltime mom, and your partner started denigrating you, belittling all you do. Or because you are no longer bringing home money, you may have begun to feel dependent on your partner. If you are a man, your partner may have become more controlling after you married or after you had children together. She may have become more secure and confident and now insists on having her way.

Whether there was a power imbalance from the beginning or it shifted over time, the fact is that you need to stop giving your power away. And in order to do this, you need to recognize the ways you give it away.

One way you may give your power away is by believing that your partner has a right to correct you or chastise you for mistakes. You must come to realize that it is not your partner's job to keep a running total of all the mistakes you make. It is not his job to correct you or instruct you on how to behave.

If something really bothers your partner, he can bring the issue to you in a respectful way, letting you know what bothers him and why and expressing how this makes him feel. If you do something that hurts him, he should feel free to tell you. But it isn't his job to tell you how you hurt someone else's feelings or offended someone else. That's their job.

Another way you may give your power away is to always ask your partner for his or her opinion on things. You may have gotten into this habit because you have a difficult time making decisions and he was always happy to make them for you. Resist this tendency to abdicate your power of choice to him and start making your own decisions. I'm not saying it will be easy because you probably doubt yourself even more now than you did in the beginning of the relationship, but after you've made a few decisions on your own, you will likely begin to trust your judgment much more and feel empowered by your efforts.

Stop Acting as If His Words Are the Absolute Truth

No matter how much he acts like the ultimate authority, the fact is that your partner is just a normal human being, no better than anyone else. Not only this, but his words are often calculated to make you feel bad—to shame you. His words are calculated to make you feel less than him, to feel inadequate, to feel unworthy of him. This is the way he can stay in charge, stay in control. Don't continue to give him that power.

When he dismisses your opinions, ideas, and suggestions, it says more about him than it does you. He does this because he either doesn't really care how you feel and what your opinion is or he is deliberately trying to make you feel small, stupid, and unimportant.

When he points out your mistakes or flaws, he isn't doing it to educate you, he's doing it to make you feel bad about yourself so he can feel superior. When he treats you like a child who needs to be managed, he is doing it because he doesn't see you as an equal partner and because he doesn't think you are as competent or smart as he is. But he is wrong. You are as competent. You are as smart. You may have different competencies than he has or you may be smarter in different areas, but you are just as competent and smart.

When he tells you that your feelings are irrational or crazy, remember that your abuser may not be capable of connecting with his true emotions, so he may actually be threatened when you are emotional. He may not be able to experience empathy toward others, so when you express concern for others, he may make fun of you. Or he may make fun of you for being "too sentimental" or "too sensitive" because he doesn't feel much at all for other people and your feelings make him feel inadequate. And he may tell you that you are overreacting or irrational because he doesn't want to face the possibility that you may be making some good points.

Stop Taking His Words and His Reactions Personally

Start listening more closely to what your partner says and when he says it. Does he tend to become more critical of you when he has been drinking? Does he start finding fault in you, in the kids, or in other relatives when he feels like a failure in other areas of his life? For example, if your partner gets passed over for a promotion, does he turn the anger he is feeling at himself on you and the kids?

Start questioning his motives and his reactions to things. Does he suddenly go into a tirade because he finds toys on the living room floor when he comes home? Instead of apologizing profusely and running to pick up the toys, stop and think a minute. Should toys on the floor really cause a grown man to lose it like this? Could it be that his anger doesn't have anything to do with the toys? Could he be angry because your neighbor just bought a new car and he is driving a ten-year-old vehicle? Could it be that he feels inadequate because he doesn't make more money? Does bullying or criticizing you make him feel better about himself? This is not a good excuse for criticizing you, but it is a good reminder that his insults have nothing to do with you and are not true.

Remember, abusers tend to take their anger out of those closest to them, especially those who they consider their property or their underlings. Instead of taking his anger or his insults personally, remind yourself that he is having problems elsewhere and with other people. If she is getting this worked up over something small, it is highly likely that she is taking her anger out on you. So don't apologize profusely, don't rush to "make it better." Just stay out of her way.

Stop Believing Her When She Tells You That Something That Seems Unreasonable Is Actually Reasonable

It is an *unreasonable expectation* that you check in with her to tell her where you are at all times, that you have sex with him every night, that you account for every penny you spend, that you cut all ties with your friends and family.

It is also unreasonable for your partner to expect that you always agree with her. Case in point, my client Zack.

> My wife expects me to always be on the same page as she is. If she doesn't like someone, she expects me to feel the same way about the person, and if I don't, she feels insulted, like I'm not supporting her in some way. If she tells me about an altercation she has had with someone, she expects me to always side with her, even when I strongly feel that she was wrong. And if she complains to me about something I've done wrong, she expects me to admit I'm wrong and to apologize, even though I feel I wasn't in the wrong at all. There is no such thing as "two sides to the story" as far as my wife is concerned, it's "my way or the highway."

Stop Believing In His Perceptions When They Seem Distorted to You

He may tell you that his perception of the way things are is the correct one, but the truth is, his perceptions are often distortions—distortions created so he will look good and you will look bad, distortions so that he never has to admit he is wrong, distortions so that he never has to look at his own issues. This is what my client Paula shared with me:

> For years I thought I was going crazy because I believed my husband's perspective about things. Even though in my gut I thought there was something wrong with his thinking, he would get so insulted if I

ever suggested that he might be wrong, that maybe he was misperceiving things, that I stopped trying. But then I began to notice that he always sees himself as the victim and he seems to only be able to see things from his perspective, never the other person's. I also noticed that this doesn't only happen with me. He'll tell me about an argument he had with someone, and it is clear that he is wrong. Even so, I dare not tell him this, or even ask him to try to see things from the other person's point of view.

Start Trusting Your Own Perceptions and Intuition

This can be an incredibly difficult thing to do since your partner's brainwashing has likely taken its toll. But if you begin to listen to your gut and start following your instincts, you can find the truth that lies there.

Gavin de Becker, author of the best-selling book *The Gift of Fear: And Other Survival Signals That Protect Us from Violence*, believes that our instinct, or intuition, can help protect us from harm if we pay attention to it. Our intuition is a sensation that appears quickly in our consciousness—noticeable enough to be acted on if we so choose—without us being fully aware of the underlying reasons for its occurrence. It is a reaction that gives us the ability to know something directly without analytic reasoning, bridging the gap between the conscious and unconscious parts of our mind, and also between instinct and reason.

Intuition is our most complex and at the same time our simplest cognitive process. It connects us to the natural world and to our own nature. As humans, we have the distinct advantage of having both instinct and reason at our disposal. According to de Becker, we are innately well equipped to make an accurate evaluation as to whether a situation or a person is safe.

Unfortunately, many of us are uncomfortable with the idea of using our instincts as a guidance tool. In fact, we spend a great deal of time ignoring or dismissing this aspect of ourselves.

This is what my client Tammy shared with me about how she began to trust her gut:

> When my husband first started complaining to me about my behavior, I trusted what he had to say. I didn't ever imagine that he might be deliberately trying to make me feel bad about myself. He always assured me it was "for my own good," and I believed him. But since I've been coming to therapy, I have begun to question the things he tells me about myself. First of all, no one else ever complains about these so-called selfish behaviors of mine. In fact, my friends have always told me that I am a generous and loving friend. Then I noticed how I felt when he complained to me. I could be having a perfectly fine day, but as soon as he starts in on me I can feel my body getting tense, like it is bracing for an attack. And when he tells me about something I've done or said that was wrong, I get this sick feeling in my stomach. It used to be that the sick feeling was all about being told about another one of my faults, but now it is because my gut is trying to tell me that what he is saying is wrong.

Begin the Deprogramming Process

Those who are being emotionally abused have been brainwashed to believe the abuser's lies, projections, and gaslighting. Therefore, you need to be deprogrammed. Just as a member of a cult needs to be deprogrammed in order to completely disconnect from the cult and its beliefs, you need to deprogram yourself of the lies and distortions the abuser has planted. This is important because unless you complete this step, your partner's lies will continue to circle around in your head and keep you mentally trapped, even long after your relationship with the abuser has ended.

This deprogramming always involves *identifying the lies* you have been told and recognizing them as the manipulation tools that they are. The following questions will help you expose your partner's lies.

EXPOSING YOUR PARTNER'S LIES

- Think of the number of times you have caught your partner lying. Many abusers are notorious liars. They lie in order to make themselves look better than they really are. They lie to excuse their bad behavior. They lie when they don't even need to lie.
- Notice how often your partner changes his story. Liars lie so much they can trip themselves up.
- Pay attention to when your partner gets most defensive. Is it when you have dared to call him on his lies, his misperceptions?
- Pay attention to how he acts when he is in public or when he is the company of people he wants to impress. Does he seem two-faced? Does he present one version of himself to others and another to you? Which version of him do you think is most likely a lie?
- Is your partner frequently in conflict with other people? Is he easily insulted, and does he start fights with others? If this is true, think carefully about the fact that your partner tends to be insulted by you and your behavior. Start seeing him for who he really

is—a person who demands to be respected by others, even when he doesn't necessarily deserve respect.

· Think of one of the traits or bad behaviors your partner has accused you of. Pick one that you don't completely believe yet. Now ask yourself, does my partner have this trait or bad habit himself? If so, he is likely *projecting* his faults onto you, either consciously or unconsciously

· Does your partner frequently accuse you of doing things or behaving in ways that you know he is guilty of?

· Does your partner tend to blame everyone else for his problems? Does he always view himself as the victim? Are people always "picking on him" or treating him unfairly? If this is the case, your partner may actually be lying to himself.

How to Deprogram Yourself

I recommend the following steps to help you deprogram yourself from your partner's lies and manipulation:

1. GET OUTSIDE FEEDBACK: Victims of emotional abuse tend to keep to themselves, both because their abusers tend to discourage or even prohibit close relationships outside their relationship and because they are so filled with shame they don't feel worthy of friendship or support. But if you still have some close friends and are still close to your family, begin to check out whether what the abuser is telling you about yourself is actually true—a reality check, so to speak. For example, instead of taking the abuser's word that you are selfish, ask a friend if that is how she sees you.

Instead of believing that you are flirtatious, ask family and friends if that is how they perceive you. The more outside feedback you can get, the more reality you will be able to take in. (An exception to this rule is if family members have been emotionally abusive toward you and you ended up getting involved with a partner who is a replica of an abusive parent or sibling. If this is your situation, you might get feedback from these people that is similar to what your abuser is telling you.)

2. Stop Blaming Yourself: If an abuser can cause his partner to doubt herself, to hate herself, she will be too busy to notice who has the real problem. Abusers are great at deflecting. Victims who continue to believe that they are the problem—that they are the one who is not good enough, inadequate, incompetent, broken, or unlovable—will have the most difficulty realizing that they are being emotionally abused. This is because they are looking in the wrong direction for answers. *Instead of always looking at yourself as the cause of the problem, you need to fix your gaze outside yourself, at the person with all the complaints.*

This is probably the reverse of what you tend to do. Whenever there is a problem, emotional abuse victims tend to look at themselves to discover what they have done wrong, to look for how they created the problem, to blame themselves.

3. Stop Trying to Change Yourself to Please Him: Stop examining your behavior to discover how you can change in order to please your partner. The truth is, you will never please him. He doesn't even want you to please him. He wants to have something to complain about, to blame and criticize you for. He wants evidence that you don't love him. Why? Because then all his own insecurity, his own shame, his own problems don't have to be looked at. He doesn't have to examine his own life to discover why he is so unhappy, why he feels so insecure, why he feels so bad about himself.

Whenever healthy people are troubled by something—when they are feeling anxious, frustrated, or otherwise upset—they look *inside* themselves for the answer. But people with an abusive personality do the opposite. They automatically look *outside* themselves. They look outside themselves for someone else to blame for making them feel bad.

The truth is, your partner likely feels terrible about himself. He has been so shamed and blamed himself that he can't stand himself. Beneath his swagger, his bravado, his self-righteousness is a scared, humiliated person. Someone who doesn't believe he deserves to be loved.

4. Stop Believing You Deserve to Be Abused: Even when you are finally able to admit to yourself that you are being emotionally abused, you may still believe the abusive treatment is justified. You may still believe you deserve it. But the truth is, no one deserves to be abused in any way. Nothing you have done or left undone in your life warrants the kind of treatment you have suffered. Unfortunately, when people are overwhelmed with shame, it is difficult to convince them that they don't deserve being mistreated.

The most important message of this chapter and this book is that you don't deserve to be emotionally abused. You don't deserve to be criticized, mocked, insulted, made fun of, berated, constantly questioned, put down in front of others, falsely accused, or called names, and you don't have to put up with any other emotionally abusive behavior. You are not so stupid, ugly, incompetent, or unlovable that no one else could love you or put up with you besides your partner. You are, just as we all are, an imperfect and fallible human being, and like everyone else, you have faults and you make mistakes—but that doesn't give your partner the right to treat you like you are worthless or unlovable.

Even if your parents treated you the same way as your partner does, it isn't proof that the problem is with you. It is only evidence that you have likely been shamed all your life and, because of this, you have grown accustomed to abuse and don't believe you deserve any better. But the truth is, you do deserve better. *You deserve to be loved and cherished and appreciated.*

5. STOP BELIEVING THAT YOU ARE UNLOVABLE: If your partner can't see your good qualities, there is a problem—and it isn't you. If your partner can't appreciate the good you bring to the relationship, he is blind—blinded by his own rage, his own shame, his own selfishness, his own experiences of being treated poorly by his family. He is blinded by his inability to recognize his own flaws and, instead, projects them onto you.

When we love someone, we appreciate the positive things about them and tolerate or accept the less positive things (with the exception of abuse). We know that no one is perfect, and we don't expect our partner to be. By the same token, when someone loves us, they don't expect us to be perfect. Anyone who does is being completely *unreasonable.*

I'm sure your partner has many faults and he makes plenty of mistakes. But hopefully, you don't have a need to address or criticize him for every mistake he makes or every fault he has. You have a right to expect the same from him. That is what loving someone is all about—accepting your partner for who he or she is, the good and the not so good (again, with the exception of abusive behavior).

In chapter 8, I will introduce you to the concept and practice of self-compassion. This will help you begin to love and accept yourself just as you are.

Rejecting Your Partner's Lies and Projections

Now let's help you to take some action toward pushing away your partner's lies and projections. The following exercise will be a good beginning.

Saying "No!" to the Words

- Let's begin by having you write down the most painful words or phrases your partner has said to you, words that have made you doubt yourself, words that have cut deep into your body and soul and made you hate yourself, words that have robbed you of your power, your confidence, your sense of who you really are. Examples of words my clients wrote down include: "Shut up," "Fat," "Lazy," and "Whore." Examples of phrases my clients put down include: "You are so stupid," "Can't you do anything right?" and "You are so fat I don't want to have sex with you."

- Take a good look at the words or phrases you have listed. Which do you still believe? Which have you come to realize are lies? Which of these words or phrases now make you feel enraged because you see them for what they are—lies intended to make you feel bad about yourself, lies that have encouraged you to just go along with his program, lies that were actually projections, lies that have distorted your reality so much that you are no longer certain what is true and what isn't (gaslighting).

- Circle those words or phrases that are most powerful for you—either because you are having a difficult time denouncing them or because they are so hurtful. These are the words or phrases you need to begin to banish from your vocabulary and from your mind.

- Focus on each of these negative words or phrases, and one by one say "No!" to them. For example, if one of the phrases that feels most hurtful to you is "You are so stupid," say "No!" to this phrase. You can simply say "No!" over and over as you look at this phrase, or you can create a sentence: "No! I am not stupid!" (You can do this silently to yourself or out loud.)

· Continue saying "No!" over and over to each word or phrase that you want to banish from your mind—either silently to yourself or out loud. Notice how you feel each time you say it.

Replacing Your Partner's Lies with the Truth

Focus on taking in the following truths, allowing them to nourish your mind and soul with all the things you so desperately need: validation, encouragement, comfort, understanding, and caring.

· The truth is it is not your fault.
· The truth is it is not your fault if he feels so bad about himself he has to bring you down.
· The truth is it is not your fault if he can't appreciate who you are.
· The truth is it is not your fault if he can't appreciate all you do for him.
· The truth is it is not your fault he can't take your love in.
· The truth is it is not your fault he is so insecure he has to try to possess you.
· The truth is it is not your fault he gets angry all the time.
· The truth is you deserve so much more.

Now write out your own list of truths: what is the truth and what is not your fault.

The truth is _____.

It is not my fault that _____.

You don't have to continue to be the receptacle of your partner's shame and anger. You don't have to continue to buy into the notion that you are responsible for his unhappiness. You don't have to continue to believe that you deserve to be punished. You don't have to continue to believe that you don't deserve to be loved or deserve to be happy. These are all lies.

There is nothing more powerful than the truth. Truth does indeed set us free. Uncovering your partner's lies—the lies he tells you and himself—will be one of the most effective ways for you to begin to emotionally free yourself from an abusive partner. In the next two chapters, I will provide you with more powerful strategies to help you continue to counter your abuser's lies, first inside your own head and then directly to the abuser.

CHAPTER 7

Using Your Anger to Deprogram and Empower Yourself

Grab the broom of anger and drive off the beast of fear.
—Zora Neale Hurston, *Dust Tracks on a Road*

HOPEFULLY, AT THIS POINT YOU have come to a place where you don't automatically believe everything your partner says and don't always take in his or her criticism. You have begun to recognize that, far from trying to help you by giving negative feedback and critiques, your partner's motive may be that he or she wants to make you feel insecure, inadequate, and unlovable. At the very least, you've begun to realize that you should not always believe your partner's version of things and you have begun to doubt his or her intentions at times.

The next step will be for you to begin to actively counter your partner's negative words and perceptions about you. You began this process in the last chapter with the "No!" exercise, and we will continue this process throughout the rest of the book.

A particularly effective way to counter your partner's negative words and begin to empower yourself is for you to connect with and release your anger. This chapter will help you to do this in three ways: (1) it will educate you about the benefits of releasing anger in healthy ways and provide you with helpful suggestions as to how you can go about it, (2) it will help you work past your

resistance to owning and releasing your righteous anger over having been emotionally abused, and (3) it will help you turn your
fear and helplessness and hopelessness into action.

Please note: most of the suggestions for releasing your anger in
this chapter refer to you doing so *indirectly*. Generally speaking, releasing your anger and confronting your partner are two separate
steps. I recommend that you find some safe ways to release your
pent-up anger before you attempt to directly confront your partner about his behavior. If and when you choose to confront your
partner directly, you need to have your wits about you. If you have
a lot of built-up anger that you have never released, your confrontation could turn into a shouting match or even end up in physical
violence. If, on the other hand, you release some of your pent-up
anger before confronting your partner, you will be able to get your
point across easier and stay on point better. I will be providing you
suggestions for safe anger release throughout this chapter.

The Many Benefits of Anger

Connecting with your righteous anger (anger that you have a right
to) is an important step in the deprogramming process. Anger can
help you push away your partner's hurtful and abusive words and
actions. Used constructively, anger can help you restore your lost
self-esteem and sense of self. Most important, anger can help you
restore your sense of power and control over your own life. There
are many benefits to expressing our anger, including:

- It is empowering.
- It can help rid you of your shame.
- It can help clear you of toxic emotions.
- It can be a motivating force.

Let's focus on each of these benefits in depth.

Anger Is Empowering

It is highly likely that you have a great deal of stored up anger toward your partner. You have probably been carrying around this anger for a long time, whether you were consciously admitting to yourself that you were being abused or not. You may have been *suppressing* your anger (consciously putting your anger aside) or *repressing* your anger (denying to yourself that you are angry). Either way, this pent-up anger has likely been sapping your energy for a long time. One of the reasons why it is important to begin to release your stored-up anger is that by doing so you will feel energized and empowered.

Unlike what you may have been taught or what you have experienced in others, anger can be a very positive emotion. Anger warns us that there is a problem or a potential threat. At the same time, it energizes us to face the problem or meet the threat and provides us with the power to overcome the obstacle. So anger is both a warning system and a survival mechanism.

Our first reaction to a perceived threat is fear. When we are faced with a threat to our survival, our nervous system prepares us to meet that threat by raising our defenses. This built-in defense mechanism is found in the sympathetic branch of the autonomic nervous system and is triggered by the release of the hormone *adrenaline*. Adrenaline helps by giving us an energetic boost, which in turn provides us with added strength and endurance to fight off our enemy or added speed in which to flee our enemy.

Although you may not have actually been in a life-or-death struggle with your partner, you have often felt threatened by his or her behavior or remarks, and therefore you have experienced a threat to your emotional well-being.

In addition to feeling threatened when someone hurts or insults us by saying something inappropriate, disrespectful, or vicious, we also become righteously angry. Unfortunately, it seldom feels safe for someone who is being emotionally abused to allow himself or herself to acknowledge that anger, much less express it. But that may be changing. If you have come to doubt your partner's negative feedback and especially if you no longer believe it, you are likely to feel some anger. You're angry about the fact that he has tried to convince you that you are selfish, stupid, ugly, incompetent, a bad mother, or any of the other negative labels he has put on you and encouraged you to believe. Hopefully, you feel angry that under the guise of being "helpful," he has caused you to doubt yourself. You feel angry that he has been manipulating you with lies all this time. If you have come to believe that you do not deserve to be treated the way your partner has been treating you, you will be especially angry.

If you are aware of feeling angry at the way your partner has treated you, it is important that you allow yourself to express that anger—to bring it out into the open. The reason this is so important is that anger release can be enormously empowering. In fact, it is one of the most empowering emotions we have.

When we allow ourselves to connect with and release our anger, we get in touch with our strength and our inner power. It is similar to igniting a flame inside us.

Connecting with and releasing your anger is also important because it will help you to find your voice. Specifically, anger can help you to stand up to your abuser and counter his or her words. When you speak your truth with your righteous anger, you are in a much stronger position to continue to push away your partner's abusive words.

Anger Will Help Rid You of Your Shame

Connecting with your anger will also help rid you of some of your shame. Blaming yourself for your own victimization robs you of your power, your sense of efficacy and agency, and your belief that you can, in fact, change your circumstances. *Instead of believing your abuser's words and continually blaming yourself for the abuse, you can push away his words with your anger.*

It is especially important for those who *internalized* their anger (i.e., blamed themselves) to redirect that anger toward their abuser. After all, your abuser is the appropriate target for your anger. By allowing yourself to get angry at your abuser, the vital force of anger will be moving in the right direction, *outward* instead of *inward*.

Internalizing your anger and blame not only makes you feel guilty and ashamed, it can also cause you to punish yourself with self-destructive behavior (such as alcohol or drug abuse, starving yourself, overeating, or self-mutilation with razors, knives, pins, or cigarettes). Let all that self-hatred become righteous anger toward your abuser. Stop taking your anger *out on* yourself and start taking it *out of* yourself.

Releasing your anger about having been abused will help you recognize that the abuse was not your fault. Although you may know on an *intellectual level* that you did not cause your partner to abuse you, nor did you deserve the abuse, expressing your anger at having been abused can help you come to know these truths on a much *deeper level*.

Releasing Anger Will Help Clear You of Toxic Emotions

If you don't find a safe outlet for your anger, it can cause serious problems in your life. Unexpressed anger has been linked to depression, various illnesses, guilt, and self-blame.

Speaking out loud about the things inside you that you haven't been able to express is extremely healing. Most victims of emotional abuse have learned to keep their feelings to themselves in order to avoid further abuse. But these feeling don't go away. Instead, they remain inside you, unspoken, unexpressed, yet still powerful. Unless they are finally released, they will begin to fester and rot, becoming more toxic as time goes by.

Releasing your anger in healthy ways is like opening the door to a dark, moldy basement. It can be scary to go into that darkness, and it can be overwhelming to feel the musty, damp air and smell the rancid smells. But by opening that door, you bring light into the situation. And you bring in fresh air so that all the rancid smells and toxins can waft out into the open air. Eventually, the light and the fresh air will replace all the darkness and toxicity.

Anger Can Be a Motivating Force

Anger can motivate you to make needed changes in your life. When you identify yourself as a victim of *undeserved* abuse, it is natural to feel angry about it, and that anger can become the energetic boost you need to get yourself out of an abusive situation. The more anger you release, the more powerful you feel. And you will also feel lighter for not having to carry around the heavy burden of anger, guilt, and shame. The lighter and stronger you feel, the more energy you will feel and the more motivated you will be to change your circumstances.

Anger: Negative or Positive?

Many people view anger as a negative emotion that is responsible for violence, crime, and other problems in society. But anger can be both positive and negative. When we use our anger to motivate us to make life changes, it becomes a very positive emotion. It can be positive when you use it to fuel your fury at the outrageous treatment you have endured at the hands of your abusive partner. It can be healing when you find safe ways to express it. Venting your righteous anger in healthy ways can mobilize, empower, and motivate you to become a stronger person. It can help you realize that you have more powers and abilities than you know.

Being angry uses a lot of emotional and physical energy. Releasing that angry energy can increase your ability to do positive things for yourself, including ending an emotionally abusive relationship. Interestingly, releasing anger can help some people think more rationally. Instead of being confused as to what you should do, you may become clearer as to what your next steps should be.

Anger is the opposite of shame. The more anger you can express in safe, constructive ways, the less shame you will likely feel. And anger can help you manage your fears. We cannot feel fear and anger at the same time. Anger tells our fear to go rest in the corner. It tells our fear that it is going to take over and protect us.

Anger can be a negative force, of course, such as when we take our anger out on innocent people. While anger can be a signal that something is wrong, we often do not take the time to discover exactly what the problem is. Instead, we simply go with the anger and let it out on whoever is around us. This is called *misplacing* our anger. It is quite common for victims of emotional abuse to take their anger out on those around them—including their children. But taking your anger out on your children and other innocent people not only doesn't solve the problem, it creates even more problems. It makes you no better than the abuser. In order for your anger to be empowering and constructive, it needs to be directed at the source—at your emotionally abusive partner. Please note: *you don't necessarily need to do this in person. Imagining that you are speaking to your abuser can be just as effective.*

Anger is also negative or unhealthy when you take the anger that should be directed at the person who hurt you and turn it against yourself. Let's say that your partner criticizes you or falsely accuses you of something. What do you do? Do you remain quiet, believe what she is saying about you, and begin to feel bad about yourself? Or do you get angry and tell your partner that you don't appreciate her criticism? If what she is saying isn't true, do you confront her with the truth or do you begin to doubt your own perceptions and believe her lies? If you do the latter, you are turning your anger against yourself, and this can be very unhealthy.

Internalized anger is anger that is bottled up and not expressed. If you feel anger but never show it, you internalize it—you keep it inside. This can have harmful effects, debilitating both your physical and mental health. Instead of fighting back and pushing away abusive comments and behaviors, you may internalize them.

You also internalize your partner's criticism when you blame yourself for the problems in the relationship, when you blame yourself instead of recognizing that what your partner is saying is not true.

Anger is especially negative when you turn it into debilitating shame. Debilitating shame robs you of your power, your sense of efficacy and agency, and your belief that you can, in fact, change your circumstances.

Still another unhealthy way of dealing with your anger is to bury it deep inside yourself where you can hardly find it. *Repressed* anger (anger you unconsciously bury) or *suppressed* anger (anger you put aside consciously) can cause depression and self-hatred. It can make you feel hopeless and helpless. Anger can hide out inside us for decades, primarily because it can feel like the riskiest emotion to express. This is especially true for women, who were raised to never acknowledge or express anger. It is also true for those who sense on an unconscious level that if they ever acknowledge their anger they will have to come out of denial—denial about just how deeply the emotional abuse has damaged them or how other abuse from childhood has impacted their lives.

Getting Past Your Obstacles

It is likely that you have some considerable resistance to the idea of releasing your anger. Here are some of the most common obstacles people have to the idea of releasing anger.

Obstacle #1: Shame and Self-Blame

Unfortunately, you may not have reached the point where you can acknowledge your anger, much less release it. One of the primary things you will need to do in order to get in touch with your righteous anger is to stop blaming and shaming yourself for the emotional abuse. *In order to accomplish this, you need to become very clear that you did not cause your partner to become emotionally abusive toward you and you do not deserve to be abused.*

Even if you can admit that you did not cause the abuse and do not deserve to be abused, it can be very difficult for you to continue to focus your anger outward, toward the abuser, instead of bringing it back to yourself in the form of shame and self-blame. This is true for several reasons:

- You've likely endured years of hearing your partner blame and shame you, and this has taken its toll on you. Healing from the effects of all this blaming and shaming can be a long process.
- You may be so used to taking the blame and shaming yourself that it may be an almost automatic response. You'll need to continually catch yourself in the act.
- It can be easier and less frightening to continue to blame yourself instead of facing the truth that you are being emotionally abused. Instead of facing the painful fact that you have been manipulated, conned, and lied to, it

can feel less painful to convince yourself that somehow you deserve this unacceptable behavior.

· You may be in the process of overcoming a lifetime of being blamed and shamed, so it is understandable that you will revert back to this habit from time to time.

Obstacle #2: Fear of Anger

Another reason why you may have difficulty connecting with your righteous anger and even more difficulty giving yourself permission to express it is that you are afraid of your anger. You may be afraid that if you start expressing it, you will lose control and harm someone. Those who were raised in violent households may be repulsed by any show of anger and may be so afraid of becoming like their abusive parent that they completely repress their own anger.

This was the case with my client Bonnie:

> My father was an extremely angry and abusive man. When he got angry, you never knew how bad it was going to get. He'd start by yelling at our mother and us kids, and before long, he was beating us. So I'm afraid to express my anger. I'm afraid I'll become physically abusive like my father.

If you are afraid of losing control and becoming abusive or violent if you were to really get angry and let it all out, or if you feel that anger is a disgusting thing and you don't want anything to do with it, the information and exercises offered here will hopefully help you get over these false, unrealistic, and unhealthy beliefs. And this is vitally important because becoming comfortable with your own anger is a major step toward empowerment and freedom.

Allowing yourself to feel and express your anger can take some work since you, like many victims, feel so *disempowered* and are often afraid of anger in general—your own as well as the anger of others.

If you witnessed a parent getting out of control or becoming abusive when he or she was angry, it is understandable that you might be afraid of doing the same thing if you start releasing your anger. In fact, this fear is a relatively common one among victims of emotional abuse. Many are so fearful of this that they don't allow themselves to become angry, much less express it. Others aren't sure why they are so afraid of feeling and expressing their anger. If this describes you, it may help you to complete the following sentences.

I'm afraid of releasing my anger because _____.

I'm afraid that if I release my anger _____.

A good way to deal with your fear of anger, no matter what the reason, is to start out very gradually by first admitting you are angry. The following exercise can be a good start.

ADMITTING YOUR ANGER

Complete the following sentences several times, spelling out your reasons for being angry. First say them out loud, and then write them down in a journal or notebook. Do it until no more answers come to mind.

I am angry with my partner for _____.

I am angry with my partner because _____.

This can be an empowering exercise or a frightening one. Pay attention to how you feel as you name the reasons for your anger and as you write them down in black and white.

Hopefully, you felt a sense of relief when acknowledging your anger and naming the offenses you've had to endure. For some of you, this can feel liberating and empowering.

For others, however, it may have been a difficult exercise. Even though you certainly have many good reasons to be angry, you may have felt at a loss for words; you may even have experienced a "brain freeze" in which you "forgot" how you've been mistreated or abused. Others may have felt like they were doing something wrong.

If you experienced any of these things while performing this exercise, spend some time writing about these feelings. Write about your fear of anger or your discomfort with it. Write about how you feel like you're doing something wrong.

There are many ways to safely release your anger without the fear of losing control, being punished, or being further shamed or abused. (I provide a list of ways later in the chapter.) Releasing your anger in healthy ways will not only help drown out the abuser's voice, but it also will help you to stop blaming yourself for the abuse and will empower you to stand up for yourself and for a better life.

Turning your fear into anger will help you stand up for yourself and refuse to be mistreated any longer. Turning your feelings of helplessness and hopelessness into anger will motivate you to continue to value yourself enough to say "No!" to anything or anyone that will undercut your value and worth. Turning your shame into anger will help you stop blaming yourself for your experiences of abuse and put the responsibility for it squarely at the feet of your abusers.

Obstacle #3: The Belief That Expressing Anger Is Wrong

Some people may tell you that you shouldn't express your anger because it is somehow more spiritual or moral to let your past go instead of releasing your anger. You ultimately need to be the one to decide whether this is true for you, but in my experience, our past experiences of being emotionally abused don't just go away, and I don't believe you can truly forgive until you've released your anger. In any case, let your body and emotions determine what is right for you and your healing process.

As my client Dina explained it:

> I was raised a Catholic and trained to believe we should always forgive others, no matter what they did to harm us. So every time I felt angry with my husband for the way he was treating me, I felt guilty. I prayed to God to help me to forgive him. But my anger just continued to come up. And it wasn't just anger, it was rage.
>
> I finally went to a woman's support group at a domestic violence center and was encouraged to express my rage. We practiced stomping our feet and screaming, and it felt so good! They had a punching bag there, and after watching other women get their anger out on it, I took my turn. My hands weren't strong enough, so I used the wooden dowel they had there, and I began hitting that punching bag over and over, imagining my husband's face on the bag. I could feel the amount of rage I had been holding in. I felt it streaming out of my arms and hands as I hit the punching bag over and over. Afterwards, I felt exhausted, but also incredibly relieved to no longer have all that rage inside me. And I felt invigorated. I felt stronger and more determined to do everything within my power to never let my husband abuse me again. My rage didn't all go away in that one session, of course, but after several more experiences of working with the punching bag, I felt my rage definitely subsiding. After that I found that I did feel more like forgiving my partner, but that didn't change

the fact that I knew I had to leave him. Because of the anger work, I now had the courage to do it.

WHAT ARE YOUR OBSTACLES?

Write down all your reasons for not wanting to release your anger. Maybe you are afraid of losing control; maybe you are fearful of facing other feelings, like sadness, that often lie underneath our anger. Perhaps you were raised to forgive and to never express anger. Whatever your reasons are, put them down on paper.

If you are having difficulty, think about your childhood and try to discover your reasons for being afraid of your anger or for your belief that anger is not supposed to be expressed. For example:

- Were you frightened when one or both of your parents expressed anger? Did one or both of your parents become verbally, emotionally, or physically abusive when he or she expressed anger?
- As a child, did you come to believe that anger was a precursor to someone hurting you?
- Were you given permission or encouragement to express your dislike of unfair situations, or were you given the message that you needed to keep quiet?

What If I Just Don't Feel Angry?

Some of my clients tell me that they don't feel angry at their abusive partner, even after they have come to realize they have been abused. These are some of the reasons clients have given for not feeling angry:

- "I don't feel angry at my husband for the way he treated me. I'm more angry at myself for putting up with it."
- "I don't feel angry at my partner. I know she didn't mean to be abusive toward me. She's apologized to me many times, and I know she's trying to do better."
- "I'm not angry at my husband; I feel sorry for him. He had a terrible childhood, and he's suffered because of it all his life."
- "My husband couldn't help abusing me. He learned to be abusive from his father. How can I be angry for him doing what he was taught?"

Do you relate to any of these comments? If not, write down your own reasons for not feeling angry at your partner for abusing you.

The first reason on the above list is unfortunately a common one. Victims of emotional abuse tend to blame themselves for putting up with the abuse far more than they blame their partner for being abusive. This "blaming the victim" mentality runs rampant in our culture. Victims of abuse are viewed as masochists or as weak or stupid. We see this attitude when a woman is raped ("It's her own fault, she was drinking too much"), we see it with physical abuse ("Why would a woman put up with this? There must be something wrong with her"), and yes, we see it with emotional abuse ("Why doesn't she just tell him to stop treating her like that?").

Most people don't want to recognize that someone can truly be victimized—that someone can attack them out of the blue, for no reason, and they can have absolutely nothing to do with it. The reason people think like this is that it protects them from feeling vulnerable to an attack themselves. If they convince themselves that victims caused their own attack—that they either did something to cause it or they didn't do what was necessary to prevent it—they can feel safer in their own lives. *But the truth is, victims are never responsible for an attack—whether it is sexual, physical, or emotional. It is always the attacker's complete responsibility.*

We've also discussed why it can be easier to blame and chastise yourself for putting up with the abuse for so long instead of blaming and getting angry at your abuser *for abusing you for so long.* Think about what your reasons for doing this really are.

My client Rebecca had been having a difficult time admitting that she was angry at her emotionally abusive husband. She kept making excuses for him, kept telling me that he was an alcoholic and didn't even know what he had done. But avoiding her anger wasn't getting Rebecca anywhere in terms of her recovery. She remained passive in her relationship with her husband and couldn't find the courage and strength to leave him.

I suspected that the main reason Rebecca was resisting connecting with her anger was that she didn't want to connect with the pain underneath her denial. She didn't want to connect with the reality that her husband, whom she still loved dearly, had betrayed her and taken advantage of her in many ways.

While the reasons listed for not being angry may make sense and may have some truth to them, they don't preclude you from being angry at your partner. Yes, your partner may have been abused as a child, yes, he or she may have had a horrible childhood, and yes, he or she may feel bad about abusing you. *But—and this is important—you can have compassion and understanding as to why your partner is abusive and be angry at the same time.* And just because your partner is remorseful for what he or she has done to you doesn't mean it erases all your anger. Remember: you have a right to your anger, and releasing it is an extremely healthy and empowering thing to do. If you are worried about your partner's feelings, it is important to know that *there are ways to release your anger without your partner being involved and without him or her ever knowing about it.* As noted before, I offer some of these safe ways to express your anger later in the chapter.

Finding Hidden Anger

Some people just don't find it easy to connect with their anger, even when they know they "should" be feeling it. If this is your situation, here are some suggestions that might help you.

- On the occasion that you do feel angry, notice where your body holds anger. Is your jaw tight? Do you clench your jaw or grind your teeth? Do you tend to clench your hands into fists? Are your muscles tight? Now see if there are times when you don't consciously feel angry, but you're experiencing at least one of these things. These body signals are telling you that even though you might not be aware of your anger, it is there, hiding in your body. Common places where anger can hide out are our backs, shoulders, jaws, and hands. Check out your body. Do you have pain or tension in your back, shoulders, hands, or jaw? Could this be anger?
- Notice if you are often irritated with others around you. This can also be an indication that you are angry without realizing it. Being consistently irritated, frustrated, or impatient with others is a sign that you are feeling a low level of anger almost all the time.
- Notice if you are often angry or impatient with yourself. Do you have a powerful inner critic who is constantly finding fault in the things you do? Are you consistently disappointed in yourself? These are signs that you are, in fact, angry and that your anger is not really at yourself.
- Often, admitting to ourselves or others that we are angry is so frightening or so forbidden that we couch our anger

using other terms. For example, instead of saying we are angry, we say we are *frustrated* or *impatient*. Think of some of the words you use to avoid saying you are angry.

· We often take our anger out on others rather than the abuser. For example, abused partners frequently take their anger out on their children. Who do you take your anger out on?

· If you still can't find your anger, ask yourself, "What if my partner treated someone I love—my parents, my children—the way he or she has treated me?" Would you feel angry about this? Most people admit that, yes, they would be angry if someone treated their children in the ways their partner treated them. If this is your situation, why aren't you angry that your partner treats you in these ways?

· Write down all the ways you believe the emotional abuse has affected you. Does seeing these effects in black and white make you feel angry? If not, ask yourself why this is.

PRIMING THE PUMP

Even if you are not aware that you are angry about having been a victim of emotional abuse, believe me, you are. It may be buried deep inside and covered over with fear or shame, but it is there. Doing the following exercise can be like priming the pump, in the sense that it might touch off your buried or hidden anger.

First, find a private place where you won't be disturbed and where you will feel free to make noises without disturbing others or drawing attention to yourself. Ideal places can be your home (if no one is within earshot) or in your car (if you can drive to a secluded area).

As you did in chapter 5, think of one of the worst things your partner said to you or did to you. Say "No!" out loud while you continue to think about how you were mistreated. Gradually increase the volume when you say "No!" until you are yelling "No!" at the top of your lungs. Let yourself really feel your "No!" Let your voice get louder and louder.

Now think of specific things you would like to say to your partner to express your righteous anger. For example:

- "Don't talk to me in that way!"
- "What you are saying is not true! You are lying."
- "I don't believe you anymore!"
- "No, I don't want to!"
- "Get away from me!"
- "I hate you!"

Repeat the phrase you chose out loud—over and over. Let your voice get louder and louder. Don't hold back; let yourself express your righteous anger. If a memory comes up, go with it and use it to fuel your anger and rage. *Please note: If you have a memory or a flashback of being yelled at or physically abused, try hard to turn the tables on the abuser.* You be the one who is yelling or hitting. Above all, don't remain in the position of being the victim. If this continues, stop the exercise.

If you get in touch with some deep, unexpressed anger—brava! That's what we're aiming for. Notice how it feels to release this anger. If you really let yourself go and you yelled loudly and for a long time, you might end up feeling exhausted, but you may also feel a sense of relief. If you start to feel scared of your anger, remind yourself that you are safe and that you are not hurting anyone. If releasing your anger uncovers more pain, let the tears flow. Tears don't weaken or diminish your anger—or power.

Healthy Strategies for Releasing Anger

In this section, I suggest healthy strategies and exercises to help you connect with and vent your righteous anger—anger that will empower you to stop taking in the negative messages and shame that the abuser bombards you with, anger that will empower you to decide that you are no longer willing to put up with abusive behavior, and ultimately, anger that will motivate you to end an abusive relationship if that is what you decide you need to do.

Consider any or all of the following, depending on what seems most appealing to you:

- Write down your angry feelings. Don't hold back; let all your feelings of anger and hurt come out on the page. Write a letter to your abuser that you do not intend to send. Let him know how the abuse affected you.
- Walk around your house (assuming you are alone) and talk out loud to yourself, expressing all the angry feelings you are having. Don't censor yourself; say exactly what you want to say to your abusive partner. Examples: "I hate the way you talk to me!" "Don't expect me to be nice to you or have sex with you after you've treated me so horribly!" "Stop taking all your anger and shame out on me!" or "Get the hell away from me!"
- Imagine you are facing your abuser as he sits in a chair across from you and tell him exactly how you feel about what he did to you. Don't hold back and don't censor yourself. If you notice that you are afraid to confront your abuser in this way, imagine that he is tied to the chair. If you don't want to see his eyes for fear of becoming intimidated, imagine that he is blindfolded. And if you are afraid of what he might say to you in response to your anger, imagine that he is gagged.
- Put your head in a pillow and scream.

- If you feel like you need to release your anger physically, ask your body what it needs to do. You might get the sense that you need to hit, kick, push, break things, or tear things up. Honor that intuitive feeling by finding a way to release your anger in a safe, but satisfying way. For example, it is safe to kneel down next to your bed and hit the bed with your fists. If you are alone and no one is around, you can let out sounds as you hit. You can lay on your bed and kick your legs, or you can stomp on egg cartons or other packaging. You can rip up old clothes or go to a deserted place and throw rocks or bottles.

Note: some researchers and some therapists believe that it isn't healthy to reinforce angry and violent behaviors (such as hitting your bed with a tennis racket, hitting a punching bag, or yelling). If you have a history of being violent, like hitting, pushing, or kicking people, I encourage you to release your anger in other ways, such as writing down your feelings or using art to express your rage. But for most victims, expressing their anger, even doing so physically, doesn't make them violent. Instead, it empowers them to say "No!" and to be more assertive, especially with their abusive partner. It also helps them release years of pent-up anger—anger they never before felt they had permission to express. Since most victims did not get the chance to express their feelings of anger when they were being abused or assaulted, doing so now is extremely healthy.

Notice how you feel after releasing your anger in any of these ways. As my client Teresa expressed to me, "I noticed that my rage felt cleansing. Like it burned away my shame and self-blame. I noticed that I had more and more energy the more I released my anger."

Releasing your anger, in addition to empowering you, also will help you recognize that any emotional abuse you've suffered was not your fault and that you didn't deserve the abuse. Although you may know on an *intellectual* level that you did not cause your partner to emotionally abuse you, expressing your anger at having been abused can help you to come to know these truths on a much deeper level. In expressing your righteous anger, you will be drowning out the voices of shame inside you.

If you are still having difficulty giving yourself permission to get angry or fear that you will lose control if you get angry, please refer to my book *Honor Your Anger*.

A Warning about Confronting the Abuser

This chapter has been about the positive aspects of acknowledging and expressing your anger at having been abused. But all the strategies and exercises are focused on *indirect* expressions of anger that don't involve your partner. If you feel like confronting your partner directly, I encourage you to continue releasing your anger in healthy, constructive ways first so that you do not put yourself or your partner at risk. I offer specific suggestions for confronting your partner about his or her abusive behavior in chapter 10.

You have a right to your anger. Let it cleanse you, heal you, motivate you, and empower you.

CHAPTER 8

Give Yourself the Gift
of Self-Compassion

*A moment of self-compassion...can change your entire
day. A string of such moments can change the course of
your life.*

—CHRISTOPHER K. GERMER,
The Mindful Path to Self-Compassion

YOU ARE PROBABLY VERY GOOD at putting yourself in your partner's
position and imagining how he feels. And you no doubt have a
great deal of compassion for how difficult your partner's life has
been and what struggles and challenges he faces every day. But I
doubt that you offer yourself the same compassion. Instead of
being concerned about your own life and your own struggles, you
probably tend to ignore these things. Instead of acknowledging
how much you suffer due to the disrespectful, hurtful, and abusive behavior of your partner, you probably minimize and deny it.
Instead of offering yourself respect and understanding for the
ways you have had to learn to cope with the abuse, you are likely
to be extremely self-critical.

My hope is that together we can turn this dynamic around,
that we can get you to be as compassionate toward yourself as
you are toward others—especially your partner. In this chapter, I
will introduce you to the concept and practice of self-compassion

and explain how it can aid you in healing from the emotional abuse you have experienced, as well as help you gain the courage, strength, and determination to end an abusive relationship.

The word *compassion* comes from the Latin roots *com* ("with") and *pati* ("suffer"); in other words, it means to "suffer with." Whereas compassion is the ability to feel and connect with the suffering of another human being, self-compassion is the ability to feel and connect with *your own suffering*. More specifically, for our purposes, self-compassion is the act of extending compassion to yourself in instances of suffering or perceived inadequacy and failure.

Kristin Neff, a professor of psychology at the University of Texas at Austin, is the leading researcher in the growing field of self-compassion. In her groundbreaking book, *Self-Compassion: The Proven Power of Being Kind to Yourself*, she defines self-compassion as "being open to and moved by one's own suffering, experiencing feelings of caring and kindness toward oneself, taking an understanding, nonjudgmental attitude toward one's inadequacies and failures, and recognizing that one's experience is part of the common human experience."

Providing yourself with self-compassion is going to be the most healing thing you can do for yourself. Primarily, it will help you to be less critical and impatient with yourself—a habit you no doubt have taken on due to the amount of criticism you have heard from your partner. It will help you judge yourself less harshly and move you toward more *self-acceptance*—something you desperately need.

Think of yourself as a cactus that lives in the harshest conditions—little water, extreme heat, few nutrients from the sand you are planted in. Even under these sparse conditions you have managed to survive, but certainly not to thrive. I want you to thrive. I want you to be one of those cacti that bloom beautiful pink flowers.

The way for you to do this is with self-compassion. Providing yourself with self-compassion will be like having a soft rain pour down on you, satisfying your thirsty soul. It will be like a gentle wind coming up to cool your parched skin. And most important, it will be like precious nutrients sinking into your hungry spirit.

Self-compassion begins with acknowledging your suffering. If you don't do this, you can't expect yourself to heal from the multitude of wounds you have experienced. If you are like most people, you've become accustomed to ignoring your pain and suffering. You believe you just need to "grin and bear it." *But now you need to stop and address your suffering because you can't heal what you don't acknowledge.*

Write About Your Pain

Please take the time to identify and acknowledge all the pain you have felt due to your partner's abusiveness. You've already listed all the ways he or she has been abusive to you, so now we are going to go one step further. I want you to identify and connect with the pain attached to each type of emotional abuse or each incident of emotional abuse. Here are some examples of what I am talking about:

"When my husband criticizes me, I feel pain in the following ways: _____."

"When my wife makes fun of me in front of others, it affects me in the following ways: _____."

"When my partner accuses me of things I didn't do, I feel hurt because _____."

Please take the time to connect with and then write about the pain you feel when your partner emotionally abuses you. If you haven't already bought a journal, I encourage you to do this now. Writing about your pain may be your first entry.

While you no doubt feel other emotions, such as shame and fear and anger, for now, focus on your pain. Write about the pain you feel due to your partner's treatment of you.

Here is an example of what one client wrote:

> When my partner criticizes me, I feel this intense pain. It feels like I'm being burnt with a hot iron or a hot branding tool. The hot pain pierces my skin, my organs, down to my very essence. I feel mortally wounded. The pain is so bad I can't believe I can survive it.

And here is another client example:

> When my husband starts in on me, I feel like I'm drowning. As he barrages me with one criticism after another, I feel like I'm sinking deeper and deeper. I can't breathe, and I can't stop myself from sinking. I feel helpless and hopeless.

And yet another:

> I feel absolutely overpowered by my wife's distorted logic. I can't explain myself to her, I can't help her to see reality. It is absolutely hopeless. I feel flattened by it, like someone just drove a giant steam roller over me.

These remarks give us a real sense of what it feels like to be emotionally abused. While the feeling can be different from person to person, the overall idea is the same. The pain is almost unbearable, and it has a visceral effect—a felt sense.

Your pain doesn't go away because you ignore it. Like our other emotions, we hold our unexpressed emotions inside, and these emotions can fester and grow. Offering yourself self-compassion is like reaching inside and bringing out the pain, examining it, and then cradling it in the palm of your hand and whispering softly to it:

"I see you."

"I hear you."

"I'm so sorry you have suffered."

TALKING TO YOUR PAIN AND SUFFERING

1. Sit quietly with no distractions around you.
2. Take some deep breaths.
3. See if you can find your pain by either visualizing it or noticing it in your body. You can imagine it to be an object, a color, or a shape.
4. Imagine you are reaching inside and pulling out your pain.
5. Imagine that you are placing your pain in the palm of your hand, then lift your palm up to your lips.
6. Whisper these words to your pain and suffering:

   "I see you."

   "I hear you."

   "I'm so sorry you have suffered."

Once you have begun to acknowledge your pain and suffering, you have taken the first step toward offering yourself self-compassion. Most victims of emotional abuse have received very little, if any, compassion or empathy for the suffering they have endured due to emotional abuse. Emotional abusers are notorious for lacking the ability to have empathy or compassion for others. And since most abusers are bent on blaming their partners and trying to make them feel bad about themselves, they aren't likely to express any feelings of concern, caring, or understanding of their partners' feelings. In fact, they are more likely to try to talk their partners out of their feelings and to accuse them of exaggerating, trying to get attention, or expecting too much. Victims, on the other hand, are so busy blaming and shaming themselves that they seldom if ever experience compassion for themselves. And as we've discussed, victims seldom tell anyone about the fact that they are being abused, so they miss opportunities for others to provide them with empathy and compassion.

Having self-compassion, connecting to one's own suffering, is a way of *validating* yourself, your feelings, your perception, and your experience. The emotional abuse you have experienced has done terrible things to you. It has damaged your self-esteem and self-confidence. It has made you feel so bad about yourself that you feel unworthy and unlovable. It probably has caused you to question your perceptions and even your sanity. These and other consequences of emotional abuse are some of the ways you have suffered at the hands of your partner. You need to acknowledge these wounds in order to heal them. If, on the other hand, you continue to minimize or deny how you have been harmed by your partner, not only will you not have the opportunity to heal your wounds, but you also will be adding to them day after day. Each criticism, each joke at your expense, each gaslighting experience, each unreasonable expectation, will not only create a new cut but also a deepening of old wounds.

Let It Sink In

Think about how difficult it has been for you to have to live through the emotional onslaughts you've suffered. Ask yourself: *Have I taken the time to acknowledge my own suffering?* Or have you tried to just put it away—out of sight and out of mind?

I want you to take time now to let it really sink in: the pain, shame, and fear you are faced with every day. If you start to feel overwhelmed by your feelings, you can back off and work on facing them a little at a time. Allow yourself to feel compassion for what you have endured and for what you will likely continue to endure. Acknowledge how hard it has been to be constantly criticized, threatened, yelled at, lied to, blamed, ignored, and dismissed. Acknowledge all the pain you have endured due to the emotional abuse you've suffered.

YOUR EXPERIENCES OF ABUSE

In chapter 3, I asked you to make a list of all the ways you have been abused by your partner. I'd like you to use that same list for this exercise.

- Read through your list carefully, taking time to take in the fact that you suffered from each type of emotional abuse. *Now read each item and take a deep breath.* This will allow you to absorb the fact that you suffered from this form of abuse. Do this with each and every item on your list.
- Allow yourself to experience whatever feelings arise in you. Don't hold back. Acknowledging your feelings is a major part of addressing your suffering. Once again, you don't need to do this all at once. In fact, you may only be able to address one item on your list at a time.

If you don't stop to acknowledge just how bad it really is, you run the risk of *normalizing* your partner's abusive behavior. You need to acknowledge how much the criticism, the gaslighting, the unreasonable expectations, and the constant blaming, shaming, and humiliation damages you on a daily basis. You need to admit the truth—that all of it is bad and that you don't deserve any of it.

In order for you to come to believe that you deserve to be treated with respect by others, particularly your partner, you need to learn how to recognize and then tend to your own suffering. And before you can teach others to treat you with kindness and respect, you will need to learn to treat yourself with kindness and respect. This brings us to the next step.

Self-Kindness

Once you have begun to acknowledge your suffering, you are ready to learn how to provide yourself with *self-kindness*—an important component of self-compassion. Self-compassion encourages you to begin to treat yourself and talk to yourself with the same kindness, caring, and compassion you would show a good friend or a beloved child.

If you fall down and scrape your knee, you know that you need to cleanse the wound and apply medicine to it in order for it to heal. We need to tend to our emotional wounds, too, but time after time, victims of emotional abuse get hurt by their partners and instead of taking care of the wound, they minimize how much it hurts or they ignore it completely. Left untended in this way, your wounds begin to fester and get worse. Giving yourself compassion, in contrast, is like applying a healing salve to your emotional wounds.

Unfortunately, even if you are willing to acknowledge your wound, you may not know how to apply the soothing salve of compassion to it. This will help: think about the most compassionate person you have known—someone who has been kind, understanding, and supportive of you. It may have been a parent, a teacher, a friend, or perhaps a friend's parent. Think about how this person conveyed his or her compassion toward you and how you felt in this person's presence. If you can't think of someone in your life who has been compassionate toward you, think of a compassionate public figure or even a fictional character from a book, film, or television. Now imagine that you have the ability to become as compassionate toward yourself as this person has been toward you (or as you imagine this person would be toward you). How would you treat yourself? What kinds of words would you use when you talk to yourself?

This is the goal of self-compassion: to treat yourself in the same way the most compassionate person you know would treat you—to talk to yourself in the same loving, kind, and supportive ways that this compassionate person would talk to you.

SELF-COMPASSIONATE WORDS

1. Say or write down something that expresses compassion toward yourself for each item on your list of ways your partner has abused you. Do this as if someone outside yourself is saying the words. For example, "I'm so sorry your wife said those horrible things to you. They were not true, and she had no right to hurt you like that," or, "It must have been so confusing for your partner to constantly lie to you like that and try to make you feel like you were crazy. That should have never happened to you. I'm so sorry." If you can't think of something to say to yourself, think of what a supportive friend or family member might say if you told him or her about how your partner abused you. Take all the time you need with this.

2. Now think about the entirety of everything you have been through with your partner—all the pain, all the suffering. Say to yourself (out loud or silently) the words that will most comfort you. *The*

words you most long to hear. Again, if you experience difficulty, it might help if you imagine
someone who has been kind and loving toward you
saying the words. If words don't come to mind, say
things to yourself like:

- "I'm so sorry your partner treats you in this way."
- "No one should have to endure treatment like
  that."
- "Oh, how horrible. That must have been so pain-
  ful, so humiliating."
- "I'm sorry you've had to endure this all alone."

3. Put your arms around your shoulders or across
   your stomach, as if someone is hugging you. Let
   yourself feel comforted. Get a cup of hot tea and sit
   quietly, letting it all sink in—all the pain, all the humiliation. Let your tears flow if you feel sad. Know
   that the way you have been treated is not okay.

Think about how much the abuse has damaged your self-
confidence, self-esteem, and self-concept, how much it has
caused you to blame yourself and even hate yourself, how
much it has affected your ability to trust, to obtain and maintain a healthy relationship, to experience a fulfilling sexual life.
Give yourself credit for how hard you have to work just to
maintain your sanity. This acknowledgment and compassion
for all you've suffered is what will help you to gain the strength
and courage to do what is best for yourself, to put yourself
first, to believe that you deserve a better life than this.

You've just offered yourself self-compassion. It isn't a complicated process to learn. It is just about acknowledging your
suffering and attending to that suffering. It is just about treating yourself with the same kindness, understanding, and care
you would give to a wounded loved one.

Compassion: The Antidote to Shame

Another benefit of learning how to practice self-compassion is that it is the antidote to shame. I think I've made it clear that the most damaging effect of emotional abuse is shame. Therefore, we need to focus on helping you to rid yourself of this debilitating shame in order for you to begin to heal from the emotional abuse you have suffered.

You need to offer yourself the healing benefits of self-compassion in order to rid yourself of the overwhelming shame you likely feel due to having been emotionally violated and feeling out of control; the shame you feel because you can't stand up for yourself; the shame you feel because you have taken in your partner's criticism and complaints and have come to believe you are stupid, ugly, incompetent, a bad mother, a lousy wife; the shame you feel at being blamed for your own abuse; and most important, the shame you feel because you have come to blame yourself.

In this chapter and moving forward, I will offer various self-compassion tools and strategies to help you decrease or eliminate the shame that you have experienced due to the emotional abuse you have suffered, as well as the shame that may have plagued you for your entire life.

By following the strategies outlined here, you can begin to rid yourself of the belief that you are worthless, defective, bad, or unlovable. Instead of trying to ignore these false yet powerful beliefs, instead of denying your shame and the feelings it engenders, you need to bring your shame out into the light of day.

Recent research into the neurobiology of compassion as it relates to shame has revealed new information about the neural plasticity of the brain—the capacity of our brains to grow new neurons and new synaptic connections. According to these studies, we can proactively repair and replace old shame memories with new experiences of self-empathy and self-compassion.

Countering Your Partner's Critical and Shaming Voice

An important aspect of the deprogramming process is for you to begin to replace the shaming and the abusive lies and accusations of your abuser with a more nurturing inner voice. As stated earlier, shaming words can worm their way into the minds of abuse victims, causing you to endlessly hear your abuser's critical voice in your head. In this section, we will focus on ways to drown out these critical messages and replace them with more nurturing and empowering words.

Let's begin by helping you become aware of how often you replay your abuser's negative, shaming messages in your head. The following exercise will help you start.

YOUR ABUSER'S CRITICAL MESSAGES

1. Begin by noticing how often you hear critical messages inside your head.
2. Notice whether these messages are the words your partner has spoken to you. For example: "You're stupid." "You can't do anything right." "No one else would put up with your shit." "You're too sensitive."
3. Now notice if the critical messages in your head are the result of the way your partner has treated you: "I must not be loveable." "I'm a terrible partner." "My feelings aren't important."
4. Begin making a list of the critical or shaming words and phrases you hear. For example, my client Robin wrote this list:
   - "Why can't you do anything right?"
   - "Why are you so stupid?"
   - "I don't know why I ever married you."

- "You're the coldest fish I ever met."
5. Notice when these messages tend to rear their ugly heads. For example: when you make a mistake, when you attempt something new, when you have accomplished something, or when someone has given you a compliment.
6. Now notice how you have made your partner's shaming words and criticisms your own—how he no longer needs to say them because you are now saying them to yourself.

The next step is to counter the critical or shaming messages in your head. The next time you hear your partner's words as he is chastising you about something you did or did not do, counter this negativity by telling yourself something like:

- "I'm doing the best I can."
- "I think I did a great job. Maybe your expectations are too high."
- "I'm just fine the way I am."
- "I want you to stop criticizing me all the time."
- "If you stopped abusing me, I'd feel more loving toward you."

When you say something like, "I'm doing the best I can," it is not the same as making excuses for your behavior; it is just a compassionate acknowledgment that we all can sometimes fail, even when we try our hardest.

The next step is to begin to replace your partner's critical or shaming voice with another voice—a nurturing inner voice. The following exercise will help you begin this process.

CREATING A NURTURING VOICE

1. Take a deep breath and begin to go inside yourself.

2. You may become aware of a wall of anger, sadness, fear, or guilt, or you may just feel a void inside. Tell yourself that whatever you find inside, it is okay. Continue to focus inside anyway.

3. If you notice a wall of thoughts, step over the wall and begin to sink into yourself more deeply.

4. Focus inside, and see if you can find even a fledgling sense of connection with yourself.

5. Bring up a nurturing inner voice. This is not a harsh, critical, or depriving voice, and it is not an overly sweet, indulging voice. It is a warm, kind voice that cherishes you and accepts you for who you are. In time, this voice will become your own, but for now, it can be any voice that meets your needs (for example, the voice of someone who has been kind to you or the voice of a beloved character in a film).

6. Notice what this kind, loving voice is saying.

7. If you aren't able to bring up a kind, nurturing voice, don't despair. Continue to think about someone in your life who spoke to you in a nurturing voice and remember how it felt when this person spoke to you kindly. Remember the dialogue of a kind, loving character in a book or movie, and imagine this character speaking to you in this way. The more you imagine being spoken to in a nurturing way, the more you will be able to internalize these loving messages.

Taking in Compassion from Others

Learning to practice self-compassion is not an easy task. It takes practice. It may also take receiving compassion from others. It can be especially difficult to learn to provide compassion toward yourself if you have never been the recipient of compassion. Many of you reading this book may have never received healing compassion, not even from your closest family and friends. Instead of family members showing kindness, concern, and compassion for one another, you may have only witnessed and experienced criticism, faultfinding, and complaints. For this reason, I want you to experience some compassion firsthand, from me. While I realize it can be difficult to imagine I am speaking directly to you, please try.

> *You've suffered for so long.*
> Night after night, you have cried silently to yourself
>   as you lie in your bed—feeling so alone even
>   though there is someone right beside you.
> *You've suffered for so long.*
> Feeling sad.
> Feeling guilty.
> Feeling angry.
> Feeling afraid.
> *You've suffered for so long.*
> Questioning your feelings.
> Questioning your worth.
> Questioning your sanity.
> *You've suffered for so long.*
> Feeling sick.
> Feeling exhausted.
> Feeling useless.
> Feeling defeated.
> Feeling empty.
> *You've suffered for so long.*

Feeling crazy.
Feeling like a failure.
Feeling like a fool.
I want you to know that I see your suffering.
I have great compassion for your suffering.
I'm deeply sorry that you've been so hurt.
So shamed.
So unappreciated.
So criticized.
So falsely accused.
So alone.
So unloved.
You deserve to be seen.
Appreciated.
And loved for who you are.
You are enough.
You are more than enough.

See if you can allow yourself to take in these words of support and compassion. Try to allow yourself to believe that I see you, that I see your suffering. Try to believe, as I do, that you deserve to be seen, deserve to be comforted.

Now you try giving compassion to yourself.
Acknowledge your suffering.
Acknowledge your pain.
Feel compassion for the fact that you've been abused
    for so long.
Tell yourself the words that will help to heal you—the
    words you long to hear.
Let the warmth of compassion embrace you like a
    soft, comfortable blanket.
Let it seep into your broken heart and fill up the
    empty spaces.

> Let it soothe your wounded soul.
> Let it wash away your shame and guilt like raindrops
>   on a dusty leaf.
> Let compassion cleanse you of your pain and fear
>   and leave you feeling new again.
> Free from self-doubt, self-criticism, and self-hate.

True strength, true empowerment comes from being connected to yourself—your feelings and your needs. It doesn't come from denying your feelings or becoming numb in an attempt to avoid your pain and suffering. Address your wounds; heal them with the soothing balm of compassion and learn from them. As the famous quote from Ernest Hemingway attests, "The world breaks everyone and afterward many are strong at the broken places." Be one of those who becomes stronger at the broken places.

Stop pretending to be strong. Stop denying your pain. Become truly strong with the power of self-compassion. Let yourself feel compassion for the amount of suffering you have endured due to being emotionally abused. Let self-compassion help you to heal the pain, fear, humiliation, and, most of all, shame you carry around due to the emotional abuse you have suffered, both as an adult and as a child. Let it help you learn how to be kinder to yourself and more forgiving of your shortcomings (imagined or real). This will encourage you to take better care of yourself in every situation you encounter.

MOVING FORWARD, I will continue to offer you ways to provide yourself with self-compassion. By practicing self-compassion, you will become more sensitive to your suffering regarding your interactions with your partner, as well as the suffering due to abuse experiences you might have had in your childhood. You will gain a deeper understanding of yourself and the reasons why you have put up with abusive behavior, and you will become more able to forgive yourself for not taking care of yourself better. Most important, you will grow to love and respect your-self more and become more motivated to take care of yourself and protect yourself from future harm.

In summary, practicing self-compassion can:

- Help you come out of denial about how you have suf-fered in the past.
- Provide you a way to comfort yourself and to validate your feelings.
- Help you to stop shaming and blaming yourself for things other people have done to you.
- Help you to forgive yourself for not being able to protect yourself or treat yourself well in the past.
- Help empower you to stand up for yourself. Research shows that self-compassion and empowerment are posi-tively related.

PART III

DETERMINING WHETHER YOU SHOULD STAY OR GO

CHAPTER 9

Is There Hope for Your Relationship?

False hopes are more dangerous than fears.
—J. R. R. TOLKIEN, *The Children of Hurin*

MAKING THE DECISION AS TO whether to stay in the relationship and try to make changes or to give up and end the relationship is an extremely difficult one for many victims of emotional abuse. While there are many things to focus on, there are three primary factors that you need to carefully consider in making your decision:

1. How much damage the emotional abuse has caused you and/or your children,
2. Whether your partner is an unintentional or intentional abuser, and
3. Whether your partner has a personality disorder.

The Damage

One of the most important aspects of the decision-making process is determining how much damage the emotional abuse has caused you. In addition to instilling shame, emotional abuse does extensive damage to the mental health of its victims, including causing depression, anxiety, the abuse of alcohol and drugs, and difficulty relating to others.

Depression

You may already be aware that you feel depressed a great deal of the time. If you aren't aware of this, check out the primary symptoms of depression listed below:

- Depressed mood most of the day, nearly every day
- Markedly diminished interest or pleasure in activities most of the day, nearly every day
- Changes in appetite that result in weight losses or gains unrelated to dieting
- Changes in sleep patterns
- Loss of energy or increased fatigue
- Restlessness or irritability
- Feelings of anxiety
- Feelings of worthlessness, helplessness, or hopelessness
- Inappropriate guilt
- Difficulty thinking, concentrating, or making decisions
- Thoughts of death or attempts at suicide

Although it is common for people to experience some of these symptoms at some point in their life, those who are being emotionally abused often suffer from what is referred to as *clinical or major depression*, which can often require medication to manage or treat. In order to be diagnosed with major depression, you need to experience five of the symptoms listed above for at least two consecutive weeks. In addition, at least one of the five symptoms must be either (1) depressed mood or (2) loss of interest or pleasure. If you meet these criteria, you are being severely damaged by the emotional abuse you are experiencing.

Anxiety

Many victims of emotional abuse experience intense worry, fear, and anxiety due to the abuse. They feel terrified, stressed, or on edge a great deal of the time, sometimes to the point of feeling physically ill. Some victims also feel disoriented—meaning that things seem unreal. If the level of anxiety that you experience becomes so severe that your symptoms significantly interfere with your everyday life, it may mean you have an anxiety disorder such as generalized anxiety disorder or panic disorder.

Alcohol and Substance Abuse

Abuse victims often turn to alcohol and drugs to manage the distress they feel due to the abuse. And unfortunately, many drink excessively and begin to abuse alcohol. (Moderate alcohol use includes drinking no more than two standard drinks a day, no more than four on any single occasion, with several alcohol-free days a week.)

Difficulties Relating to Others

Abuse victims often experience difficulties relating to others. This can include becoming irritable with others, particularly their children, and emotional outbursts, including outbursts of anger, often directed toward their children. They often withdraw from family and friends, stop attending social activities, become overprotective, and have difficulty expressing and managing their emotions.

PTSD and Complex PTSD

By far, the most significant damage caused by emotional abuse is post-traumatic stress disorder (PTSD) and complex post-traumatic stress disorder (C-PTSD). It is important that you become aware of these disorders and how they can affect you.

PTSD is a severe anxiety disorder with characteristic symptoms that develop after the experience of an extremely traumatic stressor. People who suffer from PTSD often relive the experience through nightmares and flashbacks, have difficulty sleeping, and feel detached and estranged, and these symptoms can be severe enough and last long enough to significantly impair a person's daily life. PTSD is marked by clear biological changes as well as psychological symptoms. It is complicated by the fact that it frequently occurs in conjunction with related disorders such as depression, substance abuse, and problems of memory and cognition.

Many victims of emotional abuse can be diagnosed with PTSD. In some cases, the symptoms can become more debilitating than the trauma. This disorder is also associated with impairment of a person's ability to function in social and family life, including inability to work, marital problems and divorces, family discord and difficulties in parenting.

Are You Suffering from PTSD?

The following questions will help you determine whether you are, in fact, suffering from PTSD as a result of the emotional abuse you are experiencing. Do you have intrusions concerning the abuse in a least one of these ways?

- Do you have repeated, distressing memories or dreams associated with the abuse?
- Do you sometimes act or feel as if the abuse is happening again (flashbacks or a sense of reliving it), even when it isn't?
- Do you experience intense physical and/or emotional distress when you are exposed to things that

remind you of the abuse? For example, something you see on TV or in a movie?

Do you avoid things that remind you of the abuse in at least one of the following ways?

- Do you avoid thoughts, feelings, or conversations about the abuse?
- Do you avoid activities and places or people who remind you of the abuse?

Since your experiences with emotional abuse began, do you have negative thoughts and moods associated with the abuse in at least two of the following ways?

- Blanking on important parts of it
- Negative beliefs about yourself, others, and the world and about the cause and consequences of the abuse
- Feeling detached from other people
- Inability to feel positive emotions
- Persistent negative emotional state?

Are you troubled by at least two of the following feelings?

- Problems sleeping
- Irritability or outbursts of anger
- Reckless or self-destructive behavior
- Problems concentrating
- Feeling "on guard"
- An exaggerated startle response?

Source: This quiz was adapted from the American Psychiatric Association's *Diagnostic and Statistical Manual of Mental Disorders, 5th Edition: DSM–5* (Arlington, VA: American Psychiatric Publishing).

When people are continually subjected to the same stressor over and over, they can develop the more severe form of PTSD known as C-PTSD. The impact of complex trauma is very different from that of a trauma resulting from a one-time or short-lived event such as a major car accident, a weather-related trauma such as an earthquake, flood, or tornado, or being the victim of a crime such as having your car stolen or your house broken into. *The effects of repeated or ongoing trauma—caused by experiences such as emotional or physical abuse—change the brain and also change the victims at a core level.* They change the way victims view the world, other people, and themselves in profound ways.

The following are some of the effects of complex trauma:

- **Hopelessness and helplessness:** Due to enduring and ongoing abuse, victims can come to believe that there is absolutely no hope of things changing or of them being able to escape the abuse.
- **Dissociation:** When abuse is ongoing, the brain uses dissociation as a coping mechanism. Dissociation can range from detachment or feeling as if one is outside of one's body, a loss of memory, and constant daydreaming or "checking out" of a situation to more life-impacting forms such as dissociative identity disorder, a disorder "characterized by a disconnection between thoughts, identity, consciousness, and memory" (according to the National Alliance on Mental Illness).
- **Suicidal thoughts:** Complex trauma victims are at a high risk for suicidal ideation (thoughts of suicide) as well as for being actively suicidal since the deep emotional pain they experience can feel unbearable. Suicidal ideation can become a way of coping since victims come to feel they have a way to end the severe pain if it becomes any worse.
- **Difficulties with emotional regulation:** It is common for victims of emotional abuse to experience intense emo-

tions—emotions that are often difficult to manage and regulate. This can include emotional outbursts and intense anger.

· **Fear of trusting people:** Those who have endured ongoing abuse, particularly from significant people in their lives, develop an intense fear of trusting others.
· **Hypervigilance:** When abuse is ongoing, many victims develop *body hypervigilance*—a phenomenon in which the body remains continually tense, as though it is bracing for potential trauma. This can lead to pain issues and chronic pain.
· **Flashbacks:** When trauma happens, the way the mind remembers an event is altered. These memory disturbances can create vivid involuntary memories that enter a person's consciousness, causing the person to reexperience the event. This happens most often with those who suffer from PTSD and C-PTSD. Flashbacks can feel as though you are actually being drawn back into a traumatic experience—like it is still happening or happening all over again. They can stir up images, sensations, and emotions of the original event, and they can provoke a similar level of stress in the body.

The above information will hopefully help you to determine the extent of the damage you have experienced and continue to experience due to the emotional abuse you have suffered.

Damage to Your Children

Research clearly shows that children who witness intimate partner abuse, including emotional abuse, are just as traumatized as those who are physically or emotionally abused themselves. So don't fool yourself into believing that your children are not being damaged by the emotional abuse. Your partner doesn't need to emotionally abuse your children directly in order for them to suffer from negative and sometimes severe consequences. For example, in 2003, a team of researchers led by Marilyn J. Kwong surveyed more than a thousand adults in Vancouver, Canada, and determined that growing up in abusive family environments can teach children that the use of violence and aggression is a viable means for dealing with interpersonal conflict. This can increase the likelihood that the cycle of violence will continue when they reach adulthood.

Whether you realize it or not, your children are being negatively affected by your partner's abuse and by your tolerance of it. The tension and hostility that exists in your home will cause your children to feel insecure, frightened, and off-balance. You may think your children are too young to understand what is being said between you and your partner, but even the youngest children know when one parent is being disrespectful, critical, or demeaning toward the other. Even the youngest children understand when one parent makes the other feel humiliated or inadequate. Older children pick up on the disrespectful, abusive attitude of one parent toward the other and feel they must take sides. They either feel anger and hatred toward the parent who is being abusive or they lose respect for the abused parent and begin to mimic the abusive one. The longer the emotional abuse continues in your relationship, the more your children will be affected.

Whether the Abuse Is Intentional or Not

Although all emotional abusers have a lot in common—in particular the strong likelihood that they were deeply shamed as a child—there are some major differences. These differences can determine whether they are willing and able to change their emotionally abusive behavior. So, another factor of extreme importance in making your decision whether to stay or end your relationship is determining whether your partner's abuse is *unintentional* or *intentional*. From my experience, I have determined that there are two major categories of abusers: the unintentional, unconscious abuser and the deliberate, conscious abuser.

While some abusive partners deliberately use words, gestures, silence, or scare tactics to manipulate or control their partner, many do so without *conscious intent*. This is particularly true when people are unconsciously repeating their parents' behavior. This doesn't, however, mean that their behavior isn't still emotionally abusive, nor is their behavior any less destructive or damaging to their partner or the relationship. *For the purpose of clarity, I wish to broaden the definition of emotional abuse to include any behavior or attitude that emotionally damages another person, regardless of whether there is conscious intent to do so.*

There is a lot being written lately about narcissism, and some books on emotional or psychological abuse insist that most abusers are narcissists. One book in particular makes the case that all psychological abusers are narcissists, sociopaths, or psychopaths and that all psychological abuse is conscious and intentional. I strongly disagree. After working with abusers and victims of emotional abuse for more than thirty years, it is my experience that while some emotionally or psychologically abusive partners are indeed narcissistic, and even sociopathic or psychopathic, many are definitely not.

Certainly, some partners deliberately and maliciously set out to destroy their partner. But some emotionally abuse their partner without conscious intent. The type of emotional abuser who is not consciously choosing to abuse has two subsets:

1. Abusers who do so because they were abused or neglected (and shamed) themselves as a child and are unconsciously repeating their parents' behavior, sometimes even repeating their parents' words.

2. The personality disordered person—most particularly the person who suffers from borderline personality disorder. The borderline personality disordered person's major defense is to create distortion in order to avoid being shamed. This person cannot tolerate shame of any kind (including admitting when he or she is wrong) and will do anything to avoid it, including lying, gaslighting, and distorting reality.

People in the first subset can and do change if motivated to do so, while those in the second subset suffer from a personality disorder that precludes them from changing on their own. They can, however, change with the right kind of professional help.

First, let's talk about the types of abusers who can change if they are motivated to do so.

The Abuser with a History of Abuse or Neglect

If your partner has a history of child abuse or neglect, it very well may be the cause of his or her abusive behavior. Put simply, a person is more likely to become abusive if he or she grew up in an abusive household. Violence is a frequently identified long-term consequence of child abuse and neglect, particularly for those who have experienced physical abuse or witnessed domestic violence. Research has also found that child maltreatment (particularly child neglect) and low family cohesion were associated with the frequency of intimate partner abuse. Specifically, studies showed that adults with documented histories of childhood neglect were at increased risk for a greater number and variety of acts of psychological abuse. Most profoundly, childhood neglect disrupts the child's attachments to parental figures, and this leads to insecure adult attachment styles and, ultimately, marital violence (emotional or physical abuse) in an attempt to control the partner and prevent threats of abandonment.

Not only is the abuse inflicted by such people unintentional, sometimes they do not even realize they are being abusive. This was the case with my client Joseph. He was raised by an aggressive, angry father and a mother who reacted to her husband's emotional abuse by retreating into alcohol abuse. Joseph felt abandoned by his mother and vowed to never be a victim like she was. Unfortunately, without realizing it, he took on the abusive characteristics of his father as a way to avoid becoming a victim.

> When my wife told me that I was emotionally abusing her, I was shocked. She described the ways I had treated her, and I believed what she was saying. But I didn't recognize the man she was describing. He didn't sound like me at all—at least not how I perceived myself. The man she was describing sounded like my father.

Unfortunately, when our first experiences of intimacy were fraught with fear, abandonment, humiliation, or smothering, we often can't help but repeat these behaviors when we become adults and enter into intimate relationships.

I am also a good example of someone who became emotionally abusive in my intimate relationships without realizing it. I grew up with an extremely critical and judgmental mother who had very strong opinions about things and was always certain that her beliefs and opinions were right. She was dismissive of other people's ideas and opinions and often made me feel foolish because of my ideas and beliefs. Although I swore I would never be like her, sadly, I repeated her behavior without realizing it. I took on the same air of authority that she did, and without realizing it, I ignored or dismissed my partners' opinions. Worse yet, I became extremely critical of them.

It is actually quite common to repeat an abusive parent's abusive behavior, even when we try our hardest to not be like him or her. Others become emotionally abusive as a way of surviving the stress of an intimate relationship. Most people initially feel loving feelings for their partner, otherwise they wouldn't have chosen to be with him or her. But those loving feelings can be destroyed by feelings of anger when their hopes are dashed—when their partner fails to meet their expectations or when they come to feel rejected, betrayed, or abandoned by their partner. To complicate things, sometimes people can become emotionally abusive because they are insecure about losing their partner, often due to abandonment issues from childhood. In such situations, their loving feelings become distorted by their feelings of insecurity and fear of abandonment. This is often the case with those who become overly controlling and overly smothering of their partner.

Still others become emotionally abusive because of their fear of intimacy. This is especially true of those who grew up with parents who were overly controlling or emotionally smothering. When such people enter an intimate relationship, they can become threatened by too much closeness and sabotage the relationship in a misguided effort to achieve some distance or separation from their partner. They may push their partner away, emotionally, physically, or sexually—often by becoming overly critical of their partner.

On the opposite end of the spectrum, we find adults who were emotionally neglected or abandoned as children. You would think that when such children grow up, they would welcome intimacy and closeness with a partner, but ironically, many find too much closeness threatening and they, like those who were smothered, do such things as find fault with their partner or pick a fight in order to gain some emotional distance. Others who were neglected or abandoned are clingy, as you would expect, exhibiting a need to control their partner for fear of losing him or her. These partners can become overly jealous and suspicious, fearing that their partner will abandon them as their parents did.

There is also a significant connection between witnessing domestic violence or emotional abuse and becoming emotionally abusive oneself. While women who grow up in violent families have been reported to be at increased risk to become victims of spousal abuse, the majority of studies report a link between family-of-origin violence and *men's* perpetration of intimate partner violence. For example, it is estimated that men who report experiencing family violence are three to ten times more likely to engage in partner violence than men without such histories.

Adults with a history of child physical abuse or witnessing domestic violence may be more likely to become abusive in their intimate relationships because they learned that such behavior is an appropriate method for responding to stress or conflict resolution. They learned to view emotional and physical violence as valid ways to vent anger and deal with their own self-perception issues and internal fears. So as adults, abusive behavior is normalized in the family, as is protecting themselves and avoiding what is painful by focusing on one's partner as the cause of one's unhappiness.

Also, being abused or witnessing abuse can destroy children's ability to trust others and can weaken their ability to control their feelings. This can produce dependent, hostile, and emotionally insecure people with a deeply weakened ability to build and maintain healthy relationships. In addition, low self-esteem, uncontrolled jealousy, and deep feelings of inferiority covered up by a false sense of superiority and entitlement can fuel abusive behavior.

Adverse consequences of childhood abuse and/or neglect, such as PTSD and the development of ineffective coping strategies, may also help to explain why childhood abuse is linked to intimate partner violence victimization and perpetration.

Abuse or Coping Mechanism?

Most of the behaviors we have discussed throughout the book are considered emotionally abusive. Even so, some of these behaviors cannot always be labeled "emotional abuse"; sometimes they are unhealthy coping mechanisms. While they can have the same effect on the partner who is the recipient of these behaviors, it is the *motivation* of the person behaving in these ways that can make all the difference.

Case in point: the silent treatment. Although the silent treatment is an unhealthy coping strategy, it is the intent of the action that is important. For example, the following are the conditions in which the silent treatment is *not intended* to be emotionally abusive:

- She withdraws from you physically and/or emotionally because she has a *fear of confrontation*. This can be due to several things, such as a fear of losing you, not knowing how to communicate her feelings, or simply because she lacks the confidence to stand up to you. This is certainly not a healthy way of solving problems because by avoiding discussing issues, she may build up resentment toward you. But her silence isn't intended to hurt you or control you.
- He withdraws as a way of taking a *"time out"* from the relationship. This is perfectly normal and often can be a positive way to resolve conflict in healthy relationships. If done to punish or hurt you, it is considered emotional abuse, but if done in a correct way and with correct intent, it can be a healthy strategy. For example, if your partner tells you he is taking a time out, that it is only temporary, and that he plans on talking it out at a later time, this is a healthy strategy, not emotional abuse.

As it is with the silent treatment, your partner may engage in emotionally abusive behavior without realizing the impact it has on you. In fact, many emotionally abusive partners are oblivious to how their negative behavior affects others around them. In chapter 10, we will discuss the potential benefits of discussing with your partner how his or her behavior hurts you if you haven't already done so.

So Can an Unintentional Abuser Change?

Since this type of abuser tends to be oblivious to the fact that he or she is being emotionally abusive, in general, the *unconscious abuser* is more likely to be willing (and able) to change once he or she becomes aware of their abusive behavior and how it affects his or her partner and/or children.

This is what my client Edward shared with me at our first session:

> I feel just terrible about what I've done to my wife. She recently told me she wanted a divorce because I've been emotionally abusing her for years. I was absolutely shocked. I didn't know what she meant by "emotional abuse," and I certainly didn't think it warranted getting a divorce over. She handed me one of your books and said, "If you really want to know what it is, read this."
>
> I read it, and I was appalled to find that I was guilty of many of the behaviors you listed in the book. Believe me when I tell you, I didn't know these behaviors were abusive. I just thought that this is the way people who are married treat one another. This is how my father treated my mother, so I thought it was normal.

Edward was motivated to change. "I'll do anything to save my marriage," he told me, and in fact, he worked very hard to change his abusive behaviors.

Since the publication of my book *The Emotionally Abusive Relationship: How to Stop Being Abused and How to Stop Abusing*, I have received many e-mails from abusive partners seeking my help. As it was with Edward, the impetus for reaching out for help was that their partner had either left them or was threatening to leave them. Although their motivation was to get their partner back rather than actually feeling repentant, many were nevertheless willing to do the work that enabled them to make important changes. So even if your partner's motivation is self-serving (to save the relationship), real changes can be made.

The Connection Between Emotional Abuse and Substance Abuse

There is also a strong correlation between emotional abuse in intimate relationships and alcohol and substance abuse. For example, intimate partner violence against women is two to four times more likely when they are with men who drink alcohol. And the American Society of Addiction Medicine states, "Victims and abusers are eleven times more likely to be involved in domestic violence incidents on days of heavy substance abuse."

It is common for a normally understanding and loving partner to become abusive whenever he or she becomes high or intoxicated. Technically, this type of emotional abuse can go under the category of unintentional abuse since the abuser is not necessarily trying to control or shame his or her partner, at least not consciously.

What he or she can be doing, albeit on an unconscious level, is dissipating his or her anger. This is where the connection between previous childhood trauma and emotional abuse can come in. There is a strong association between childhood abuse and neglect and later substance abuse in adulthood. In particular, men with child sexual abuse histories are found to be at greater risk of substance abuse problems. The higher rates of substance abuse problems among adult survivors of child abuse and neglect may, in part, be due to victims using substances to self-medicate from trauma symptoms such as anxiety, depression, and intrusive memories caused by an abusive history.

If your partner has such a history, or if you suspect that he or she does, *there may be hope for your relationship if—and I stress if—he or she is willing to seek therapy for his or her childhood trauma and/or seek help for substance abuse.*

The Personality Disordered Abuser

Another type of abuser who abuses without realizing they are harming their partner is the individual with a personality disorder. What is a personality disorder? According to the *DSM-5*, the diagnostic and statistical manual used by mental health professionals to help determine psychological diagnoses, a personality disorder is "an enduring pattern of inner experience and behavior that deviates markedly from the expectations of the individual's culture, is pervasive and inflexible [unlikely to change],...is stable over time, and leads to distress or impairment in interpersonal relationships."

In addition to an inability to have successful relationships, those with a personality disorder suffer from disturbances in self-image, ways of perceiving themselves and others, appropriateness of range of emotion, and impulse control. There are ten types of personality disorders, some of which can cause a person to exhibit behavior that can be experienced as emotionally abusive, but three personality disorders stand out from the others because those who suffer from them will almost always create an emotionally abusive environment when they are in an intimate relationship. These disorders are *borderline personality disorder (BPD), narcissistic personality disorder (NPD), and antisocial personality disorder (APD).* While other personality disorders and mental illnesses can cause a person to at times become emotionally abusive, those people with BPD, NPD, or APD tend to be, by their very nature, emotionally abusive on a regular basis.

I am singling out BPD and NPD here because they, more than any other personality disorder or mental illness, are believed to be primarily caused by emotional abuse and neglect in childhood. Another reason for my focus is that BPD and NPD are considered by many to be the personality disorders of our time. The sheer numbers of people suffering from these disorders has caused a great deal of focus on them, including a great deal of research as to their cause.

In this section, I will define and describe these two personality disorders, illustrate how each is manifested, and explain how each is experienced as emotional abuse by the other partner. I will also provide questionnaires to help you determine whether your partner may have one of these two disorders. In later chapters, I will offer concrete advice and strategies that partners can use to help them maintain their sanity and work toward eliminating the most damaging emotional abuse in the relationship.

Neither does it mean that if a person has BPD, he or she does not also have NPD. According to new research, including a study referenced in the third edition of *Stop Walking on Eggshells*, in 2008 a team of researchers interviewed 35,000 people in the community. They discovered that nearly 40 percent of the people who had BPD also had NPD. In other words, if your partner has BPD and is not currently in treatment, there is a 40 percent chance that he or she also has NPD. Therefore, I suggest you read the information below on Narcissistic Personality Disorder.

You no doubt have noticed that throughout the book I have been alternating using the male and female pronouns, but in this chapter, I will primarily use "she" when discussing borderline individuals and "he" when discussing narcissistic individuals. This doesn't mean there are no male borderlines or female narcissists, however. In fact, in recent years, professionals are finding that they are encountering more and more male borderline and female narcissistic clients.

Determining Whether Your Partner Suffers from Borderline Personality Disorder

Those involved with a partner who has BPD or who suffers from strong borderline traits often do not realize they are being emotionally abused. They may know they are unhappy in their relationship, but they may blame themselves or be confused as to what is causing the continual disruption in their relationship. They are often blamed for the relationship problems or made to feel that if they would only be more loving, more understanding, more sexual, or more exciting, their relationship would improve. The irony is that a partner of a person with BPD is actually codependent or dependent, causing him or her to be extremely patient and willing to put up with intolerable behavior.

Partly because they are constantly being blamed for things they did not do, those partners who are involved with borderline individuals often come to doubt their own perceptions or their own sanity. Often accused of behaving, thinking, or feeling in ways that upset their partner, they tend to adapt a careful style of living that authors Paul T. Mason and Randi Kreger call "walking on eggshells"—and they've written a book called *Stop Walking on Eggshells: Taking Your Life Back When Someone You Care About Has Borderline Personality Disorder*. Many people come to believe that they are not only the cause of their relationship problems but the cause of their partner's emotional problems as well.

DOES YOUR PARTNER SUFFER FROM BORDERLINE PERSONALITY DISORDER?

The following questions, adapted from *Stop Walking on Eggshells* by Mason and Kreger, will help you determine whether your partner suffers from BPD or has strong borderline traits.

1. Has your partner caused you a great deal of emotional pain and distress?
2. Have you come to feel that anything you say or do could potentially be twisted and used against you?
3. Does your partner often put you in a no-win situation?
4. Does your partner often blame you for things that aren't your fault?
5. Are you criticized and blamed for everything wrong in the relationship or everything that is wrong in your partner's life, even when it makes no logical sense?
6. Do you find yourself concealing what you think or feel because you are afraid of your partner's reaction or because it doesn't seem worth the hurt feelings or the terrible fight that will undoubtedly follow?
7. Are you the focus of intense, violent, and irrational rages, alternating with periods when your partner acts normal and loving? Do others have a difficult time believing you when you explain that this is going on?
8. Do you often feel manipulated, controlled, or lied to by your partner? Do you feel like you are the victim of emotional blackmail?
9. Do you feel like your partner sees you as either all good or all bad, with nothing in between? Does there seem to be no rational reason for the switch in her perception of you?
10. Does your partner often push you away when you are feeling close?
11. Are you afraid to ask for things in the relationship because you will be accused of being too demanding or told there is something wrong with you?

12. Does your partner tell you that your needs are not important or act in ways that indicate that this is how she feels?

13. Does your partner frequently denigrate or deny your point of view?

14. Do you feel you can never do anything right or that her expectations are constantly changing?

15. Are you frequently accused of doing things you didn't do or saying things you didn't say? Do you feel misunderstood a great deal of the time, and when you attempt to explain, does your partner not believe you?

16. Does your partner frequently criticize you or put you down?

17. When you try to leave the relationship, does your partner try to prevent you from leaving by any means possible (e.g., declarations of love, promises to change or get help, implicit or explicit threats of suicide or homicide).

18. Do you have a hard time planning activities (e.g., social engagements, vacations) because of your partner's moodiness, impulsiveness, or unpredictability? Do you make excuses for her behavior or try to convince yourself that everything is okay?

If you answered "yes" to many of these questions, your partner likely has traits associated with BPD. As you can see from this list, many of the above behaviors have already been described in this book as emotionally abusive (e.g., constant criticism, unreasonable expectations, constant chaos, emotional blackmail, gaslighting).

What you were probably unaware of was that many of these abusive behaviors are also symptoms of a personality disorder.

While it is impossible to diagnose someone without seeing her, I can say with a great deal of certainty that if your partner thinks, feels, and behaves in many of these ways, she probably suffers from BPD. For more information on the characteristics of BPD, refer to the resources recommended at the end of the book.

What causes BPD? Those who suffer from BPD or have strong borderline tendencies almost always experienced some form of abandonment when they were an infant or child. This abandonment may have been physical (e.g., the hospitalization of a parent, the death of a parent, being put up for adoption, being left in a crib for hours at a time) or emotional (e.g., having a mother who was unable to bond with her child, being an unwanted child whose mother neglected her, having a detached and unloving father). Children who were victims of sexual abuse can also feel abandoned and betrayed—especially if the perpetrator was someone they loved and trusted, such as a parent, a sibling, a grandparent, or a trusted family friend. And if they were not believed when they divulged the abuse or they came to realize or suspect they were not being protected by a loved one or someone they trusted, they can also feel abandoned. This physical or emotional abandonment causes the borderline individual to be extremely afraid of being either rejected or abandoned in an intimate relationship, which would make her feel the original wounding all over again, or to be distant and detached as a way of defending herself from the potential pain of intimacy. In many cases, the borderline individual actually vacillates from one extreme to the other. This is commonly referred to as experiencing the "twin fears of abandonment and engulfment."

For example, at one point in time a borderline individual may herself be emotionally smothering —desperately clinging to her partner, demanding a great deal of attention, begging her partner to never leave her. At another point, however, perhaps only hours or days later, the same person can be overwhelmed with the fear of being engulfed. She may become distant and withdrawn for no apparent reason, or she may push her partner away by accusing him of not loving her, of being unfaithful, of no longer finding her attractive. She may even accuse him of being too needy.

Over the course of a relationship, the most typical pattern that emerges is that a borderline individual will "fall in love" very quickly and will push for instant intimacy. She may seem to have few, if any boundaries—insisting on seeing her lover every day, sharing her deepest, darkest secrets, even pushing to marry or live together right away. But once she has captured her partner's heart and received some kind of commitment from him, a typical borderline individual may suddenly become distant or critical, or have second thoughts about the relationship. She may stop wanting to have sex, saying that she feels they had sex too early and didn't get to know one another in other ways. She may suddenly become suspicious of her partner, accusing him of using her or of being unfaithful. She may begin to find fault in everything he does and question whether she really loves him. This distancing behavior may even verge on paranoia. She may begin to listen in on her partner's phone calls, check on his background, or question past lovers. This behavior on the part of the person suffering from BPD may cause her partner to question the relationship, or it may make him so angry that he distances himself from her. When this occurs, she will suddenly feel the other fear—the fear of abandonment—and she will become needy, clingy, and "instantly intimate" once again. For some partners, this vacillation may be merely perplexing, but for many it is extremely upsetting. And in some cases, it will cause the partner to want to end the relationship. When this occurs, there will no doubt be a very dramatic scene in which the borderline individual may beg for him to stay, threaten to kill herself if he doesn't, or even threaten to kill him if he tries to leave her.

Even though many of the typical behaviors of a person suffering from BPD are clearly emotionally abusive, often the relationship becomes mutually abusive because the borderline partner pushes her partner to his limit and he ends up acting out in frustration and anger. This kind of vacillating behavior is very difficult for most people to cope with and few come away from the situation without losing their temper or resorting to abusive tactics themselves.

Determining Whether Your Partner Suffers from Narcissistic Personality Disorder

Many who suffer from NPD straddle the fence between being unintentional abusers and ones who do so intentionally. I include those who suffer from NPD here in the unintentional category for now and will explain the difference between those who abuse intentionally and those who do so unintentionally in the next chapter.

NPD includes symptoms such as poor self-identity, inability to appreciate others, sense of entitlement, lack of authenticity, need for control, intolerance of the views and opinions of others, emotional detachment, grandiosity, lack of awareness or concern regarding the impact of one's behavior, minimal emotional reciprocity, and a desperate need for approval and positive attention from others.

DOES YOUR PARTNER SUFFER FROM NARCISSISM?

1. Does your partner seem to be constantly wrapped up in himself—his interests and projects—and have little interest in what is going on with you? Even when he does take an interest, does it seem ingenuine and is it short-lived?
2. Does your partner like to be the center of attention? Does he become bored or rude when someone else has the floor? Does he tend to bring the conversation back to himself?

3. Does he seem to feel he is entitled to special treatment from you and others?

4. Does he seem to lack empathy and compassion for other people? Does he seem to have particular difficulty feeling other people's pain, even though he expects others to feel his?

5. Does your partner feel that his opinions and beliefs are always the right ones and that other people (including you) really don't know what they are talking about?

6. Does he think he is smarter, hipper, more attractive, or more talented than almost anyone else?

7. Does he seem to have an inordinate need to be right, no matter what issue is being discussed? Will he go to any lengths to prove he is right, including browbeating the other person into submission?

8. Is your partner very charismatic, charming, and/or manipulative when he wants something, only to be dismissive or cold after a person has served her purpose?

9. Have you come to distrust your partner because you have frequently caught him in exaggerations and lies? Do you sometimes even think he is a good con man?

10. Does he often appear to be aloof, arrogant, grandiose, or conceited?

11. Can he be blisteringly insulting or condescending to people, including you?

12. Is he frequently critical, belittling, or sarcastic?

13. Does your partner become enraged if he is proven wrong or when someone has the audacity to confront him on his inappropriate behavior?

14. Does he insist on being treated a certain way by others, including waiters and waitresses in restau-

     rants, store clerks, and even his own wife and children?

15. Does he frequently complain that others do not give him enough respect, recognition, or appreciation?

16. Does he constantly challenge authority or have difficulty with authority figures or with anyone who is in a position of control or power? Is he constantly critical of those in power, often insinuating that he could do better?

17. Does your partner seldom, if ever, acknowledge what you do for him or show appreciation to you?

18. Does he instead seem to find fault with almost everything you do?

19. Even when he is forced to acknowledge something you've done for him or a gift you've given him, does he somehow always downplay it or imply that it really didn't meet his standard?

20. Does your partner focus a great deal of attention on attaining wealth, recognition, popularity, or celebrity?

21. Is your partner charming and manipulative when he wants something, only to be aloof and dismissive when his needs have been satisfied?

If you answered "yes" to more than half of the above questions, your partner may be suffering from NPD or may have strong NPD traits. For more information on this disorder, refer to the next chapter and to the resources recommended at the end of the book.

So, what causes a person to become narcissistic? Personality disorders such as NPD are often created during childhood and adolescence due to a child's lack of healthy attachment to his primary caretakers. Most suffered from a lack of true attachment due to emotional neglect during childhood and their teen years. While their physical needs for food and shelter were met, they did not have their emotional needs met (such as attention or validation).

Although you may feel a great deal of compassion for a partner with such a history, you need to be careful to not let your compassion cause you to excuse his behavior. Many people, perhaps including yourself, suffer from a lack of healthy attachment to their parents due to emotional neglect. But not all victims of emotional neglect suffer from NPD. What distinguishes these individuals from others is (1) the severity of the emotional neglect, (2) a lack of corrective experiences, such as having a loving grandmother, caretaker, teacher, or other compassionate adult who provided some of the nurturing, attention, and validation they so desperately needed, (3) a decision made along the way to *"meet my own needs at any cost"* (deciding that no one was ever going to meet their needs, so they needed to meet them themselves, no matter what it took to do so), and (4) the development of an attitude of entitlement (taking on the attitude that "life owes me" for what they didn't receive in childhood). Regarding that last point, when they didn't get what they wanted or needed, they insisted on getting it and they were furious with others for not giving it to them. This included taking what they wanted, including using other people with no regard for their feelings.

Another way that a lack of true attachment can occur is through extreme and repetitive overindulgence. In these cases, the child was not taught normal societal rules but was given free rein to do whatever he wanted. There was a severe lack of boundaries or rules in the home, and often the parents gave their child the message that he was so special or talented he didn't need to follow normal rules. When a societal rule was broken, such as a child or adolescent being caught stealing, his parents typically covered up for him and no punishment was given. The overindulged child or teenager began to view others as mere vehicles to satisfy his needs.

A third cause of narcissism is to have parents or caretakers who have absolutely no conscience or shame themselves. Being raised by another narcissist, sociopath, or psychopath sets the child up to be the same. This can include parents who are always trying to fool the system, are out-and-out criminals, or were raised in societies that live outside the rule of law.

Can Someone with Borderline Personality Disorder or Narcissistic Personality Disorder Change?

A major difference between abusers with the above personality disorders and others who were neglected, overindulged, or abused in childhood is that the former experienced extreme shame in their childhood or adolescence. Because of this extreme shame, they needed to build up a wall in order to protect themselves from being further shamed through criticism or exposure.

When most survivors of abuse and neglect reach adulthood and are around other people outside the home, they notice that their behavior is not acceptable to others or they experience a great deal of pain whenever they are in an intimate relationship. Once this occurs, many seek out counseling, self-help books, or seminars in order to change what they now realize is harmful behavior. But unfortunately, those who have developed a personality disorder due to the defensive wall they have built up are usually blind to the fact that their behavior is unacceptable or even damaging to others, even when it is brought to their attention. Instead, they cling to the defensive illusion that there is nothing wrong with them. Even when they are forced to acknowledge that their behavior is unacceptable, they refuse to actually believe it. Their defenses are such that they are convinced that they are always right and that other people just don't understand them, and in this way they can protect themselves from further shame.

Even though they may not consciously become abusive in their relationships, abusive partners who suffer from personality disorders cannot readily change and are usually not motivated to do so. Even those who are willing to make changes typically need years of specialized psychotherapy in order to do so.

Nevertheless, there are some rare exceptions: people who suffer from BPD or NPD who are willing to enter psychotherapy and work hard to change. But even when such people do go into therapy, they seldom continue for long. It becomes too painful for them. And any so-called changes they make are usually short-lived. One of the main reasons for this is that they cannot or will not be self-reflective and therefore risk exposing their true self—even to themselves. It is always someone else's fault. It is always the other person who needs fixing.

Even if they lose jobs, have failed marriages, or get into legal trouble, in the end, the way those with these personality disorders choose to live their lives works for them. Even with good therapy, in which they are encouraged to become aware of how the walls they have built up to protect themselves from further shame keep them from true intimacy and how much better their life could be without those walls, most are not willing to do the work required to let down those walls.

IN MAKING YOUR decision whether to continue or end your relationship, you should keep all three of the major considerations we have discussed in mind: (1) the damage the emotional abuse is causing you and your children, (2) whether your partner is an unintentional or intentional abuser, and (3) whether your partner has a personality disorder. But by far, the most important question to ask yourself is "Is my partner willing and able to change?" You will not learn whether your partner is willing to change unless you directly let him or her know that he or she is being abusive and in what ways. In fact, confronting your partner is so important that if you can't bring yourself to do so, you need to focus more on how you can end the relationship than on saving it.

In the next chapter, we will focus specifically on how to confront your partner about his or her abusive behavior and whether it is safe or recommended that you do so.

CHAPTER 10

Confronting Your Partner

For everything that gets taken from you,
Don't let your voice be one of them.
—ANONYMOUS

I HAVE SHARED WITH YOU information on how to empower yourself and decrease your shame by countering your partner's abusive words and by practicing saying "No!" to his or her abusive behavior. And we've focused on how to offer yourself self-compassion for your suffering. Hopefully, these actions have brought you to the place where you can now confront your partner about his abusive behavior. But if you are not there yet or you can't imagine you will ever be able to confront him because you are afraid of the consequences, there is no chance that your partner will stop being abusive. *Put simply, if you can't confront your partner, if it feels too dangerous, or if you feel like you aren't strong enough to do it, you probably shouldn't consider staying with your partner.*

This doesn't mean that there is something wrong with you if you can't confront your partner. Not being able to confront him can indicate that you realize that to do so is useless (either because you've tried before or you know that your partner is generally never willing to see his faults or shortcomings) or you are afraid to do so for fear of disastrous results (i.e., you are afraid your partner will lash out in anger or will make threats against you such as taking your children away from you). In fact, it is not safe to confront a person who has been physically violent in the past.

While some of you have never confronted your partner about his abusive treatment of you, some have already spent many hours trying to understand your partner's behavior, explaining to him why you are upset or trying to figure out what went wrong in the relationship. Some of you have also discovered that trying to reason with your partner or just complaining about his behavior has not been effective. For this reason, you must begin to respond to his inappropriate or unacceptable behavior in a new way—a way that will make an impact on him. You already have a list of the ways your partner has been emotionally abusive, and hopefully, you have also written about how his behavior has affected you. Now it is time to share this information with your partner. I'm calling this a "confrontation," but it doesn't have to be hostile or challenging. You can set up your confrontation any way you choose, including where you do it and how you go about it. If you can't bring yourself to confront in person, you can write out the ways your partner has been abusive and how it has damaged you and give it to him to read.

How to Effectively Confront Your Partner

Before you confront your partner, it is important to note that abusers seldom, if ever, acknowledge their abusive behavior. Instead, he is likely to deny that he did anything wrong, accuse you of lying, or, if he does admit any wrongdoing, blame you for his actions. This could cause you to once again begin to doubt yourself. If this occurs, refer to your list of the ways he has abused you in order to come back to reality.

The following suggestions will help you confront your partner in the most effective way possible.

- I suggest that you practice or role-play what you plan to say with a friend or counselor before you attempt to confront your partner, especially if you tend to become over-whelmed, frightened, or tongue-tied when you try to speak to him. If you don't have someone to practice with, you can put an empty chair in front of you and imagine that your partner is sitting in it. This will help you get over some of your fears about confronting him and will make you more confident about what you want to say.

· Before you talk to your partner or give the information to him in written form, explain to him that you are sharing this information in an attempt to save the relationship. Some of you may also want to explain that unless he begins to make some significant changes, you will have to end the relationship. (Note: don't say this as an empty threat. If you don't really mean it, don't say it.)

· Ask your partner to hear you out before he responds to you. If he doesn't agree with this or breaks this agreement and interrupts you, it could end up in an argument, which will be extremely counterproductive. If your partner repeatedly interrupts, you can decide to end the confrontation.

· Take a deep breath before beginning your confrontation and make sure you are in the present.

· Make sure your feet are firmly planted on the ground, whether you are standing or sitting.

· Be sure to speak clearly and firmly. Hold your head up high and look directly into your partner's eyes.

There are two ways to confront: (1) you can sit down with your partner and have a talk with him about the fact that he is being inappropriate or disrespectful toward you, or (2) you can call him on his behavior or attitude the next time he is abusive. The way you choose to go about confronting your partner will have a lot to do with the status of your relationship. If you and your partner are still emotionally close a great deal of the time and are still able to communicate with one another over most issues, you may wish to let him know that you would like to have a serious discussion. This approach will be especially effective if you have not confronted him on his abusive behavior in the past. If, on the other hand, you have confronted him before and he has ignored you or insisted that you are making too much of things, then you may need to try the second approach and confront him whenever he commits the abusive behavior. This is also the best approach for couples who have grown distant and are noncommunicative.

If you are in a relatively new relationship and have begun to see warning signs of emotional or verbal abuse, a serious discussion with your partner is probably the best approach. As we've already discussed, many people are simply unaware that their behavior is abusive. If he is relatively young or has little or no experience in a long-term relationship, he may simply be repeating one or both parents' behavior without being aware of how it affects you. Even if a person has been in previous relationships, his past partners may have put up with the abuse without saying anything or may have blamed themselves for their partner's behavior, never realizing that they were being abused.

Your decision whether to choose approach number one or number two may also have to do with whether your partner is a person who has abusive behavior or is an abusive person by nature, in other words, whether his abuse is intentional or unintentional. If he simply has some bad behaviors, approach number one may work well to help him become more conscious of how his behavior affects you. But if he has an abusive personality or has a personality disorder, approach number two will work better since reasoning with him will not likely be effective.

Approach Number One—The Serious Discussion

Tell your partner that you have something important to talk to him about and that you'd like to set up a time to do so. Make sure you choose a time that is good for both of you and a time when you will not be distracted by kids, television, or the telephone. In fact, it is best to turn off the phone and other media. If he becomes curious or anxious and wants to have the talk immediately, make sure you are in the right frame of mind before giving into his request. If you are not prepared to have the talk, simply assure your partner that while the discussion is an important one, it can wait for a more appropriate time. If you feel you are unable to talk to him at all, write him a letter.

I suggest you begin by telling your partner that you have been unhappy with some of the ways he has been treating you or speaking to you. If this is the first time you've brought this up, let him know that you care about him but that the way he treats you is affecting the way you feel about him and that you are afraid it will ultimately destroy the relationship. If you have tried talking to him about this before, remind him of this. Let him know that you haven't noticed a change on his part and that this is unacceptable to you.

If he seems open to what you are saying, tell him you appreciate his willingness to work on the relationship and ask him if he'd like some examples of the kinds of behavior you are talking about. At this point, you do not need to define the behavior as *emotionally or verbally abusive*. It will be difficult enough for your partner to hear your examples without being accused of being abusive.

Don't be surprised if your partner makes excuses or becomes defensive. This is understandable. But don't allow the discussion to turn into an argument. If he begins to accuse you of making things up, imagining things, or trying to create problems where none exist, say something like the following: "What you are doing right now is an example of the kind of behavior I have been talking about. You are negating my experience and making accusations. Please stop." If he gets angry and becomes verbally abusive, say, "You are being verbally abusive. Please stop."

Tell your partner that from now on you are going to let him know when his behavior has become offensive to you and that you hope he will cooperate by being open to these reminders so that he can begin to change his behavior.

Approach Number Two—Confronting at the Time

If you choose to tell your partner by confronting her the next time she is abusive, the following suggestions will help:

- **Speak up:** The very next time your partner says something that is abusive or treats you in an emotionally abusive way, immediately say to her, "I don't want you to talk to me that way (or treat me that way). It is inconsiderate (or disrespectful). I don't deserve to be treated that way." This will no doubt get her attention. She is likely to be startled by your response and may even be at a loss for words at first. But eventually, she will likely become defensive and deny that what you are saying is true. She may tell you she didn't do any such thing or that it was something you said or did that made her say what she said or treat you as she did. If this happens, tell her that what you have shared is not up for discussion. This leads us to the next step:
- **Don't argue; just stand your ground:** If your partner defends herself by making excuses or blaming you, don't get caught up in the argument. Stand your ground by repeating the exact words you said before: "I don't want you to talk to me that way (or treat me that way). It is inconsiderate (or disrespectful). I don't deserve to be treated that way."
- **Be prepared for silence:** Instead of arguing, some partners will completely ignore you when you confront them about their behavior. This is itself disrespectful and abusive. In essence, she is saying to you, "You're not even important enough for me to listen to or respond to."

Don't let her get away with it. If she gives you the silent treatment say, "Ignoring me and giving me the silent treatment is also unacceptable (or disrespectful), and I don't appreciate it. I deserve to be heard and for my words to be honored."

· **Offer information if requested:** If your partner seems genuinely surprised by what you have said and sincerely asks you for more information about what you meant by it, by all means offer it to her. Suggest she read this book or my book *The Emotionally Abusive Relationship*, in which I not only outline what the types of emotionally abusive behavior are but also offer a program to help abusers to change.

Time will tell whether your confrontation has had an impact on your partner. Often, such confrontations enable an abusive partner to recognize the inappropriateness of her behavior and to understand that her behavior is hurtful to her partner and is having a negative effect on her relationship. When these realizations occur, people do sometimes change.

Even those who are aware that they are being abusive sometimes stop their abusive behavior when they discover that their partner realizes he is being abused, states he will no longer allow it, and seems to mean what he says. It is also possible that your partner may have been testing you to see just how much she could get away with. Many partners lose respect for their partner when he allows abuse to occur. By speaking up and letting her know you will not tolerate such behavior, you may not only stop the abusive behavior but also gain back your partner's respect. On the other hand, some people deliberately look for partners they can dominate and control or someone who will be a scapegoat for their anger. If your new partner is such a person, your confrontation will tip her off that you are not the kind of partner she is looking for and she may choose to move on. If this is the case, you are better off without her.

Whether this confrontation and your continued attempts to confront your partner's abusive behavior are effective or not, your efforts will not be in vain. By continuing to confront your partner on his or her unacceptable behavior, you will affirm in your own mind that you do not deserve to be treated in these ways. This will, in turn, help raise your self-esteem, help rid you of your shame, and help you take one step closer to ending the relationship. In the future, you will know that you can recognize emotional abuse when it occurs and that you can respond appropriately. In this regard, confrontations tend to be more beneficial for you than they are for your partner.

Next Steps

While it will be difficult for your partner to admit that he has been emotionally abusive, it is vitally important that he do so. This may be the hardest thing he ever does since he probably has a difficult time admitting when he is wrong. If he is an especially proud person—and many abusers are—he has an investment in covering up any weakness or vulnerability with a mask of bravado. This is how many abusers have learned to deal with their shame. Asking him to admit that he has been abusive will be horrendously shaming to a person who is already full of shame. However, you need to hear his admission and he needs to say it if there is any real hope of ending the abusiveness that has nearly destroyed you and the relationship.

Your partner admitting that he has been emotionally abusive will serve several purposes. First of all, it will help him to continue to come out of denial. Dealing with the fact that he's been abusive can be so painful and so shame-inducing that he may constantly be tempted to minimize the damage he's caused or talk himself out of facing up to it. Admitting it to you will make it harder for him to deny in the future.

Your partner also owes it to you to admit that he has been emotionally abusive. You've been suffering from the effects of his behavior for some time now, and you need him to validate this to you. You need to be able to stop thinking you are crazy or that you've been imagining it all along. You need him to confirm your feelings and perceptions. And in many cases, you may need confirmation so you can stop blaming yourself for all the relationship problems and for your partner's abusive behavior.

Finally, as painful as it will be to do, your partner needs to admit that he's been emotionally abusing you because he needs to take responsibility for his actions. No hedging. No minimizing. Owning up to his behavior and taking 100 percent responsibility for it will be good for his self-respect and for his soul.

On the other hand, if you experience real change on your partner's part, you may not feel you need him to admit his abusiveness to you. This is up to you. For some, observing their partner making a real effort to stop being abusive is enough. This is especially true for those who know their partner well enough to know he is absolutely too proud to admit his faults.

Note: even though you may be tempted, please don't rub your partner's nose in the fact that he has been emotionally abusive and don't deliberately try to make him feel like a monster. Allow your partner some time to get to a place where he can finally admit his abusive behavior.

A Meaningful Apology

Many of you may feel that in addition to your partner admitting he has been abusive or making obvious changes, you also need an apology in order to continue the relationship. I recommend this if possible because it will be healing for both of you. Encourage your partner to take his time getting to the place where he can do so. A meaningful apology consists of what I call the three R's of apology—*regret, responsibility, and remedy*. Unless all three of these elements are present, you will sense that something is missing and you will feel shortchanged. Let's take a look at each element in more detail:

REGRET — A Statement of Regret for Having Caused the Hurt and Damage to the Other Person: This includes an expression of empathy toward you, including an acknowledgment of the hurt and damage that he caused you.

RESPONSIBILITY — An Acceptance of Responsibility for His Actions: This means not blaming anyone else for what he did and not making excuses for his actions but instead accepting full responsibility.

REMEDY — A Statement of His Willingness to Take Action to Remedy the Situation: He can do this by promising not to repeat the action, promising to work toward not making the same mistake again, stating how he is going to remedy the situation (e.g., go to therapy), and/or making restitution for the damages he caused (e.g., paying for your therapy).

CONFRONTING YOUR PARTNER will probably be one of the hardest things you ever have to do. But you owe it to yourself and your children to do so. If you aren't ready to confront him, I suggest you enter therapy so you can continue to work on getting strong enough to do so. If you can't afford therapy, please contact your local women's clinic or battered women's organization or your local community counseling center and ask for referrals to low-cost or no-cost therapy or inquire as to whether they offer a support group for emotionally abused partners.

If you are able to confront your partner and you discover that he or she is unaware of his or her abusiveness, and if he or she can make some connection between his or her past (i.e., the way he or she was raised) and their present behavior and is willing to acknowledge how he or she has been abusive and how it has damaged you, there certainly is hope for your relationship.

In the next chapter, we will focus on the signs that you definitely need to end the relationship or work toward doing so.

CHAPTER 11

Indications That You Need
to End the Relationship

You gain strength, courage and confidence by every experience in which you really stop to look fear in the face. You are able to say to yourself, "I have lived through this horror. I can take the next thing that comes along." You must do the thing you think you cannot do.

—ELEANOR ROOSEVELT, *You Learn by Living*

IN THIS CHAPTER, WE WILL discuss deal breakers—indications that you must end your relationship—as well as the types of abusers who are unable or unwilling to change.

Deal Breakers

If any of the following circumstances exist in your relationship, it is absolutely essential that you end your relationship as soon as possible:

· **Your children are being emotionally, physically, or sexually abused by your partner:** The truth is that it is rare for emotional abusers to confine their criticism and controlling behavior to their partner. A person who is critical, demanding, rejecting, and difficult to please generally treats everyone in his life in a similar way, especially those closest to him. Don't continue to be blind to the way your partner treats your children or to make excuses for his behavior. If you can't walk away from the abuse, get professional help. Therapy will help you continue to heal your shame and build up your self-esteem still further so you can gain the courage to do what you know is right for you and your children. You are probably who you are today primarily because of the way your parents (or other caretakers) treated you. Don't continue the cycle of abuse by exposing your children to the same unacceptable behavior you grew up with.

· **Most important,** if your children are being *physically* or *sexually abused* by your partner, it is vital that you get them away from him immediately, even if this means you have your children go stay with family or friends. Each day your children are exposed to such violence, irreparable harm is being done to their mind, body, and spirit.

· **You are witnessing the damage the emotional abuse is doing to your children:** Not only are they being damaged in the present by witnessing abusive behavior, but you also are providing them poor role models and setting them up to be either victims or abusers. Many children who become bullies or victims of bullies in school witnessed emotional or physical abuse in their own homes. If one of your children is exhibiting bullying or abusive behavior toward his or her siblings or classmates, this is a giant red flag that your child is being negatively affected by your relationship with your partner. The same is true if one or more of your children are exhibiting victim-like behavior—being unable to stand up for themselves or becoming more and more passive. Unless you and your partner are actively working on stopping the abuse, such as each of you working with a professional therapist, you are sacrificing the emotional health of your children by choosing to stay together.

· **You have become emotionally, physically, or sexually abusive toward your children:** If, as a result of being emotionally abused by your partner, you have begun to take your anger, shame, and pain out on your own children, you need to find a way to stop abusing them. The most effective way will be for you to get away from your partner. If you can't leave your partner yet, the most loving thing you can do for your children is to separate yourself from them for their protection. You can send your children to live with friends or relatives (as long as one of them isn't the same person who abused you as a child) while you get professional help. Believe me, you will earn their respect and gratitude when they learn why you did this.

· **Your partner is physically abusing you or is threatening to do so:** Many abusers start out by emotionally abusing their partner and work their way up to physical abuse. The more he is allowed to emotionally abuse you, the more permission he has to become physically abusive. If he has already hit you, even if it was "just a slap," you are in danger. The same holds true of behaviors such as pushing, shoving, pinning you down, or holding you captive against your will. All of these behaviors indicate that your partner has lost control of himself, and they are danger signs for you. In some cases, it may indicate that your partner has become mentally unstable. Don't fool yourself. If he has become violent with you once, he will do it again, and the next time it will be worse. Don't accept the excuse that he was drunk or high. He hit you because he has a problem. Drinking or using drugs may exacerbate his problem, but they are not excuses. Neither should you allow your partner to use the excuse that he has an emotional problem such as BPD. While it is true that those with this disorder can become out of control and physically violent, this is still no excuse. He needs to take responsibility for his behavior by seeking the professional help he needs. If your partner refuses to seek professional help, I advise you to separate from him until he does so. Otherwise, every day you stay in this relationship you are endangering your emotional and physical well-being, and possibly your very life.

· **You have reached a point where you are becoming physically abusive:** If you have become so frustrated and angry that you have begun to act out your anger in a physical way that could result in seriously hurting your partner or pushing him into hurting you, it's time to leave. Even if you "only slapped or pushed" your partner, unless you get professional help, you are putting your partner in more danger as each day goes by. It is important that you not only end the relationship but also seek psychotherapy to help you heal the damage you've experienced at the hands of your partner. If you honestly feel that you are not an abusive person by nature but that your partner has pushed you into becoming violent, then the best thing for both of you is for you to end the relationship. Even if your partner suffers from a mental or emotional disorder of some kind, you are not helping either of you by staying.

· **You have begun to fantasize about harming or killing your partner:** If you have reached this point, you feel trapped and believe there is no way out of your abusive relationship. But the reality is that there is a way out. You may need to get professional help in order to gain the courage and strength to leave, or if you are afraid for your physical safety, you may need to contact the police or go to a battered woman's shelter. In either case, you need to realize that there is certainly a better way out than risking being in prison for the rest of your life or being overwhelmed with guilt for the rest of your life because of the physical harm you caused your partner.

· **You are seriously questioning your sanity:** If your partner is using gaslighting techniques on you and you are beginning to distrust your own perceptions, it is time to end the relationship. The longer you stay, the more you will doubt yourself and your sanity, the harder it will be to leave, and the more your mental health will be jeopardized.

The Best Reason to End the Relationship

All the above are good reasons to leave. But the best reason of all is if your partner falls under the category of an *intentional* or *conscious* abuser. Unlike the person who abuses because this is what he learned from his family or other traumatic situations or because he believes that his behavior is normal, this type of abuser has been deliberately attempting to control you and destroy you. And because his behavior is conscious and deliberate, there is little chance that he will stop abusing you. This is because, unlike the unintentional abuser, *he wants to hurt you.*

The intentional or conscious abuser can be divided into the two subsets:

1. **The controller:** This type of intentional or conscious abuser deliberately sets out to control and shame his partner. The controller behaves, just as the name implies, in controlling, dominating ways that are considered extremely abusive. He is manipulative and controlling in both overt and covert ways. He intentionally behaves in intimidating and unpredictable ways in order to keep the victim "under his thumb" or "in her place." His abu-

sive tactics send signals to the victim that she is inferior or unworthy of respect and love from the abusive partner. Eventually, the victim is made dependent on the partner as she loses trust in herself. This brainwashing makes her feel extremely fearful, helpless, and insecure.

2. **The shameless person:** This person is often considered to have an abusive personality or to suffer from either NPD or APD. While we can all be guilty of wanting to hurt our partner when we have been hurt, a shameless partner intentionally hurts his partner on a regular basis. The shameless abuser deliberately employs emotionally abusive tactics in order to gain power and control over his victim as a way of compensating for his deep feelings of insecurity and inadequacy.

The main differences between the controller and the shameless person are the degree of emotional disturbance and the intensity of the need to harm the partner. The controller doesn't necessarily want to harm his partner. He wants to control her because he is so insecure. Controlling his partner makes him feel powerful. And he is afraid that if his partner has too much independence, she will leave him, become unfaithful, or lose interest in him.

The shameless person, on the other hand, deliberately sets out to harm and even destroy his partner for any real or imagined hurt she may have caused him. He has no limits as to what he will do, and he has absolutely no empathy or compassion for his partner— or anyone else for that matter. He also has no guilt or remorse for his actions.

Can Someone in the Intentional Category Change?

Both the controller and the shameless person are not likely to change or even be willing to change. They typically have serious psychological problems (such as NPD) that need years of therapy in order to overcome. And while people cannot help the fact that they have NPD, choosing to remain disordered and to not address their issues is something they are responsible for.

The reason a controller is not likely to change is that it would require him to let go of his need to be in total control of his partner. Since controlling others is his primary way of compensating for his insecurities, those insecurities would have to be healed or eliminated in order for any real change to occur. Controllers are not likely to allow themselves to become vulnerable enough to get the psychological help they would need in order to heal these wounds.

A major reason why there is so little hope for recovery for shameless people is that they refuse to admit that anything is their fault. They will adamantly deny that their actions are hurtful. They also tend to create the illusion that they are always right. So confronting a shameless person about his emotionally abusive behavior is usually fruitless. You can spend hours and hours trying to explain to him exactly what he has done to hurt you, to no avail. He may even acknowledge that his actions are hurtful or even harmful in the moment, only to deny the same action later on. The truth is, shameless people will never take lasting responsibility for their behaviors.

One reason for shameless people's reluctance to admit fault of any kind is that they already know what they are doing. In fact, they are choosing to continue to be abusive. Another reason why they don't admit fault is that they cannot tolerate viewing themselves as wrong or making a mistake. Still another reason why it is not likely that a shameless abuser will change is that those who fall into this category, including sociopaths and psychopaths, have an intense lack of empathy. So while they may agree to stop a certain behavior, they don't truly understand how their behavior harms other people, so they don't have the motivation to continue extinguishing the behavior. And because they have no empathy for you, they don't really care how you feel.

The shameless people who don't have the ability or the willingness to change fall into two categories: malignant narcissists and sociopaths.

Malignant Narcissism

Malignant narcissism is considered the darker side of NPD. With a malignant narcissist, expressions of aggression, antisocial behaviors, and suspiciousness are as prominent as the typical attributes of narcissism, such as poor sense of self, fragility, and egocentricity. Abuse by a malignant narcissist definitely falls under the intentional abuse category. It is also very often malevolent abuse. Malevolent abuse is abuse that is not only intentional but also deliberately undermining. This form of intentional abuse is far more insidious and far more damaging than typical emotional abuse. If your partner is bent on undermining or even destroying you, if he or she is so angry or envious or so full of hate toward you that he or she deliberately and maliciously sets out to sabotage your success, health, or happiness, he or she may be a malignant narcissist.

Malignant narcissism is a pathological syndrome composed of an extreme mix of narcissism, antisocial behavior, aggression, and sadism. Many consider it a hybrid or blending of NPD and APD. Grandiose and always ready to raise hostility levels, malignant narcissists undermine families and organizations in which they are involved and dehumanize the people with whom they associate.

The definition (according to Dictionary.com) of malignant is "disposed to cause harm, suffering, or distress deliberately; feeling or showing ill will or hatred." Those who are hurt the most by malignant narcissists are the people who love or depend on them. Family, coworkers, and employees have to walk on eggshells to appease their fragile egos and minimize the occurrence of their unstable, impulsive, or aggressive behaviors. Malignant narcissists lash out or humiliate others for even the smallest infractions (e.g., you dared to venture an opinion that differed from theirs; you demonstrated confidence, and it made them look bad; you told a joke that they took personally).

For some malignant narcissists, their grandiosity and their need to protect their fragile "true self" can be extreme, as can their lying. This can create problems for those close to them because this behavior can easily veer into gaslighting. Many of these people will become angered if their lies are challenged with truth or facts.

Those who interact with malignant narcissists often experience them as jealous, petty, thin-skinned, punitive, hateful, cunning, and angry. Given their shallowness, they cannot regulate their emotions, and they have beliefs that swing from one extreme to the other. These characteristics, coupled with the combination of poor empathy, aggression, hypersensitivity, and suspiciousness, can bring a great deal of pain to others.

Below are the traits most closely associated with malignant narcissism. Please note that no two personalities are the same and that some characteristics might appear more prominent than others, according to the individual.

- **Sadism:** Sadists gain enjoyment from the pain, suffering, and humiliation of others. They willingly inflict suffering in order to gratify themselves and to control others.
- **Proactive manipulation:** All narcissists manipulate to some degree as a way of getting what they want, but there are different types of manipulators: those who are opportunists, who take advantage of anyone in a vulnerable state, and those who are proactive in their manipulation, meaning they don't wait for an opportunity, they create it. Malignant narcissists are the latter. They get almost as much enjoyment from manipulating others as they do from making them suffer. They are also more forceful and less subtle in how they manipulate others, and they employ a great number of tactics, from

gaslighting to lovebombing. Their acts of manipulation are planned, calculated, and honed over years of use.

· **Antisocial behaviors:** Given that malignant narcissism crosses into APD territory, it is not surprising that these narcissists engage in various types of antisocial behavior. For example, they are often pathological liars, they steal and cheat, and they are prone to volatile moods, aggression, and unprovoked hostility. They are up for a fight—with anyone at any time.

· **Hypersensitivity to criticism:** While some sufferers of NPD on the lower end of the continuum can brush off criticism (after all, they are perfect and what you are saying is ludicrous), if you criticize malignant narcissists it is at your peril. They find any form of criticism an affront to their character and will go on attack at the slightest hint of it. This is because their sense of self is so fragile that it is easily damaged, and retaliation or escalation is the only way they know how to feel better about themselves.

· **Paranoia:** Malignant narcissists don't trust anyone. They are overly suspicious of everyone and believe everyone is out to get them. Because they are always manipulating others for their personal gain, they assume everyone else is doing the same. Their paranoia can lead to a state of hypervigilance in which they are always on the lookout for threats. Their preoccupation with what other people are doing can lead to them controlling the movements of their victims for fear of what they might otherwise do or say.

While they likely possess all of the traditional traits of narcissism, those suffering from malignant narcissism will also have more exaggerated narcissistic tendencies than other narcissists, particularly in areas involving harming others, aggression, and manipulation. This includes:

- **Lack of empathy:** Although all narcissists lack empathy, the malignant narcissist carries it to an extreme. Not only does he happily inflict pain and suffering on others, but he also ignores and invalidates any emotions shown by another person. While the less dangerous narcissist may be able to experience some empathy and even remorse and regret on some level, he is often unwilling to allow it to influence him. The malignant narcissist, on the other hand, simply cannot put himself in other people's shoes or relate to their feelings at all. It is a totally foreign concept to him. He also cannot feel or show any remorse for any suffering he causes.

- **Failure to accept responsibility:** While malignant narcissists may sometimes accept that they acted in a certain way, they will warp the truth to make it seem like *they were justified in doing so*. They will externalize the responsibility to someone or something else. (In other words, they will play the blame game.) More often, they will refuse to accept that their actions were wrong or unacceptable and will flat out deny responsibility for hurting others or other undesirable outcomes they have caused.

- **Envy:** Because malignant narcissists hold themselves in such high regard, when they encounter someone with a trait or lifestyle or possession they covet, they are consumed with envy. They absolutely hate to see someone with something they do not possess. As a way of coping with this, they belittle the person and/or insist it was pure luck that they obtained something. Rarely, if ever, do they acknowledge that someone deserves what he or she possesses. Instead, they are likely to attempt to sabotage someone's success in any way possible (e.g., giving bad advice, deliberately smearing that person's reputation). They revel in the failure of others, both overtly and covertly.

· **An extreme need for attention:** All narcissists need what
   are called "narcissistic supplies," including frequent attention, adoration, and affection from others in order to
   make themselves feel good and to restore their energy
   levels. But while a low-level or moderate narcissist may
   seek out more positive forms of attention (such as praise
   for a job well done or a compliment on how great he
   looks) to bolster his self-worth, a malignant narcissist
   may get almost as much satisfaction from negative attention. He may enjoy playing the villain since he is not
   afraid of confrontation and fighting. (This trait is one
   where there is less overlap with someone who suffers
   from APD or psychopathy, who typically doesn't care
   what other people think and will sometimes prefer to be
   a loner rather than the center of attention.)

All of the above qualities describe a more extreme, abusive,
and dangerous type of narcissist and one who should be avoided
at all costs.

Please note: malignant narcissism is not recognized as a separate disorder by the psychiatric profession. It is a hypothetical,
experimental diagnostic category. NPD is found in the *DSM-5*,
while malignant narcissism is not.

Antisocial Personality Disorder

In addition to the malignant narcissist, there is another type of
abuser that you should get away from as soon as possible: the person who suffers from antisocial personality disorder (APD).
Sometimes called sociopathy, this is a mental condition in which
a person consistently shows no regard for right and wrong and ignores the rights and feelings of others. People with APD tend to

antagonize, manipulate, or treat others harshly or with callous indifference. They show no guilt or remorse for their behavior—thus, they fall under my general category of being shameless.

Individuals with APD often violate the law, becoming criminals. They may lie, behave violently or impulsively, and have problems with drug or alcohol abuse. Because of these characteristics, people with this disorder typically can't fulfill responsibilities related to family, work, or school.

Symptoms of APD include:

- Disregard for right and wrong
- Persistent lying or deceit to exploit others
- Being callous, cynical, and disrespectful of others
- Using charm or wit to manipulate others for personal gain or personal pleasure
- Arrogance, a sense of superiority, and being extremely opinionated
- Recurring problems with the law, including criminal behavior
- Repeatedly violating the rights of others through intimidation and dishonesty
- Impulsiveness or failure to plan ahead
- Hostility, significant irritability, agitation, aggression, or violence
- Lack of empathy for others and lack of remorse about harming others
- Unnecessary risk-taking or dangerous behavior with no regard for the safety of self and others
- Poor or abusive relationships
- Failure to consider the negative consequences of behavior or learn from them
- Being consistently irresponsible and repeatedly failing to fulfill work or financial obligations

If your partner has some or all of the symptoms of a malignant narcissist or someone with APD, you must seriously consider ending the relationship. Someone with these disorders is not going to be able to change, even if he or she were willing to do so (and most aren't). There is absolutely nothing you can do to change this person, and you and your children are in more and more danger the longer you stay with him or her. If you aren't in the place emotionally, physically, or financially to leave this person, I strongly urge you to seek psychotherapy. You are in danger.

Please note: while those who suffer from BPD and NPD cannot or will not change without professional help, those who suffer from malignant narcissism or APD are considered unreachable, even by professional psychotherapists. Even though BPD and NPD are serious disorders, those who suffer from them are not generally beyond help.

It can be incredibly painful to face the truth that you absolutely must end your relationship, even if you still love your partner and whether you want to or not. But the sad truth is, there are times when you must do something in order to save your sanity or even your life, when you must step up and do the right thing for your children and yourself, and this is one of those times.

CHAPTER 12

If You Decide to Stay

Love yourself enough to set boundaries.... You teach people how to treat you by deciding what you will and won't accept.

—ANNA TAYLOR

SOMETIMES, NO MATTER HOW MUCH you realize that your relationship is damaging you and your children, no matter how much you come to realize that your partner is unlikely to change, you may still not be prepared to end the relationship. If this is the case, I want you to know I understand. You just may not be in the right space emotionally, physically, financially, or spiritually to make this kind of significant change in your life. I do not want to shame you any further than you've already been shamed by telling you that you are wrong for staying. But I do urge you to continue reading this book for more information on how to rid yourself of the shame that has likely put you in this situation in the first place. (You may want to skip the next chapter.) I also highly recommend that you seek counseling if you haven't already done so. A positive counseling experience will help you to continue healing your shame and prepare you to end the relationship if and when you choose to do so.

How to Proceed to Try to Make Changes in Your Relationship

If your partner has a history of childhood abuse or neglect or of witnessing domestic violence, and if he or she is willing to go into therapy in order to heal from the trauma, it may be worth it to stay and work on the relationship. There would, however, be a number of conditions that need to be in place.

1. First of all, don't confuse the fact that some abusers are not deliberately trying to control, shame, or destroy you with giving them an excuse for their behavior. Even though they may have been unaware of their abusive behavior, they are still responsible for it and for changing these negative behaviors. In other words, you can feel compassionate and understanding about why your partner is the way he is, but this doesn't give him a free pass. If he wants you to remain in the relationship, he must do everything possible to make significant changes in the way he treats you. "I can't help it" cannot be an excuse for abusive behavior. Know that you can feel compassionate toward your partner and hold him accountable at the same time.

2. You need to be able to explain to your partner exactly which behaviors of his are emotionally abusive and how these behaviors affect you. Your partner needs to *listen to you carefully, without interrupting, without making excuses.* If he can't listen openly to what you have to say, there is no hope for change. Put simply, he needs to *listen* and *learn.*

3. As a show of good faith, your partner needs to sit down with you to talk about a plan of action, including a plan for his recovery. This most certainly includes psychotherapy, since he needs to begin to acknowledge and

heal his wounds from childhood (especially his shame) in order to make any real changes. In particular, your partner needs to find a therapist to help him explore the wounds from his childhood and discover the patterns of violence, neglect, or abandonment he is repeating. He may also need to learn how to have more empathy for others, especially you. This can be a byproduct of good therapy. If your partner is suffering from an addiction to drugs, alcohol, gambling, sex, or any other compulsive or addictive behavior, he needs to treat this symptom as well. This may include attending twelve-step meetings, or it may include a stay at a recovery center.

4. If your partner has an "anger problem," you may think he needs to go to anger management classes. But while he can learn some helpful strategies to manage his anger, he really needs to learn to manage his shame. Because in reality, *anger problems are really shame problems.* Some victims of childhood abuse or neglect learned to substitute the emotion of rage in order to avoid the overwhelming feelings of shame that occurred when they were being abused, neglected, or abandoned. Instead of feeling the helplessness and humiliation that usually come with being victimized, some people learned to cover up these more vulnerable feelings with rage. This substitution of rage for shame became a habit so that anytime they feel humiliated, embarrassed, or ridiculed and their self-esteem takes a drop, they use rage to cut off these bad feelings. Good therapy will help an abusive person feel safe enough to become vulnerable, to allow feelings of shame and humiliation to surface, and to learn how to manage these more delicate feelings.

5. Abusive people also need to learn what their specific triggers are—in other words, what sets them off. Common triggers for abusive people include feeling rejected,

feeling impotent or helpless, and feeling disrespected. Once they are aware of their triggers, they need to learn to pay attention to their body and emotions so they can recognize when they have been triggered and address their true feelings instead of automatically going to rage.

6. Your plan may also include such things as your partner staying away from friends who encourage his drinking and/or drug use, or even staying away from toxic relatives who may trigger his negative behavior (e.g., every time he is around his father, he comes home angry and takes his anger out on you and the kids).

Will Counseling Help?

Most experts agree that marital or couple's counseling is not recommended for those in an emotionally abusive relationship. First, and most important, most abusers can be so charming that they often win over the therapist into seeing the relationship from their perspective. And because those who are being abused can seldom speak up for themselves, especially in the presence of their abusive partner, the only person's perspective the therapist gets to hear is the abuser's. Therefore, I recommend that you seek individual therapy for yourself and that you ask your partner to get his own therapist.

Equally important, I suggest that you consider joining a group for those who are being emotionally abused. The support you will receive in this kind of setting will be invaluable, and most victims are in desperate need of emotional support and validation. Participating in a group will also help you feel less isolated, a real problem for victims of emotional abuse. *The less isolated you are and the more support you receive, the less shame you will feel and the less you will blame yourself for the abuse.* Even an online group is better than not being involved in a group at all.

Ineffective Versus Effective Communication

Although I want to make it clear that the abuse is never your fault, it can be important to learn which types of communication are counterproductive when dealing with an abusive person and which types are more effective. For example, the following are counterproductive methods of engaging with an abusive person:

- **Appeasing:** This is an attempt to "calm down" or "keep the peace," and it is probably how you have been communicating with your partner for a long time. But instead of it being effective (meaning that your partner hears you and makes an effort to change), it is very likely that she sees your efforts as weakness, thus inviting more abuse.
- **Pleading:** Most abusers, especially those who are narcissists, have disdain for weakness of any kind (in others and themselves), thus they will not respect any efforts to improve the relationship if pleading is involved.
- **Arguing or fighting back:** This is not only futile, but it also often escalates into a major fight. While assertiveness is certainly something you want to learn and practice, arguing is not necessarily about being assertive. Being assertive is naming the offensive behavior or offensive words at the time. Once you have done this, there is no need for further discussion and certainly no need to argue. State your case and walk away.
- **Trying to get the abuser to understand you:** This is typically futile since many abusers (especially narcissists) simply don't care enough about others to want to understand them. Also, many abusers feel misunderstood themselves and are much more bent on communicating their point of view than in hearing yours.
- **Criticizing and complaining:** It is important to remember that as much as the abuser likes to criticize you

or complain about you, she is very insecure and has a great deal of shame and cannot tolerate being criticized in any way. It may seem difficult to distinguish between criticizing and calling your partner on her abusive behavior at the time. The key difference is your intent. When you criticize or complain, it is usually when you are angry and hurt and you want to make your partner feel bad in return. Calling her on her abusive behavior should be done, as much as possible, with a clear head and not for the purpose of getting back at her for hurting you.

· **Threatening:** Threatening to leave or file for divorce will not work unless you really intend to do so. The more you threaten and then do not follow through, the weaker your threats will become.

As you can see, there doesn't seem to be much left to try in order to communicate effectively with an abusive person. In fact, the only way that is sometimes effective is to be as direct and honest as you can be about what is acceptable behavior and what is not and then to call your partner on his or her unacceptable behavior at the time. Please be clear: this method typically only works with the type of abuser who seems to be abusing unintentionally (i.e., he or she is unconsciously repeating his or her parents' behavior).

Also, note that some strategies are more or less effective depending on whether your partner has a personality disorder and which type of personality disorder it is. For example, begging and pleading with a narcissist is counterproductive since narcissists have disdain for weakness and vulnerability (in others and themselves). Showing weakness to a narcissist is like adding fuel to the fire. It will encourage her to shame and humiliate you even more.

On the other hand, *validation* is an important communication tool when dealing with someone suffering from BPD who doggedly holds on to her perceptions, no matter how distorted they are. Instead of arguing with this type of person, what she really needs is to feel heard. So letting her know that you heard her and that you understand her feelings can be a powerful strategy to end the ceaseless accusations, at least for the time being. Even if you disagree strongly with what she is saying, tell her something like "I understand what you are saying and I will think about it" or "I'm sorry you are hurting" rather than continuing to argue with her, which is likely to only cause her to become more and more upset. Please refer to the recommended reading list at the back of the book for books on how to communicate with someone who has BPD.

Effective strategies for communicating with an abusive partner include:

- **Know what your boundaries are and enforce them:** Establishing healthy boundaries can help you feel stronger and less overwhelmed, so decide which behaviors you are willing to accept and which you are not. For example, you may be willing to accept his preoccupation with himself and his rudeness but not be willing to tolerate his name-calling. You don't need to give a reason or explanation, but you do need to follow through. If you have told him, "If you continue to call me names I will end our conversation," then do so if he continues. Don't wait for his reaction, and don't engage with him no matter what he says or does. The more quickly and decisively you act, the better. Just get up and walk away. Your partner will try to argue with you or convince you that you are overreacting or treating him unfairly. He will try a number of approaches to see if he can induce guilt or confuse and intimidate you. No matter what he tries, remember: your boundaries are not up for discussion. (Know ahead of time that once you set healthy boundaries, narcissists, in particular, will likely escalate their attacks or threaten to end the relationship.)

- **Consider which of his behaviors are most upsetting to you:** Which ones cause you the most pain or confusion? These will be the behaviors you need to speak up about the most.
- **Include consequences when setting your boundaries:** You need to decide what you are prepared to do if your boundaries are ignored or violated. Your consequences need to be clear in your mind ahead of time so you don't have to figure them out in the moment. You need to only communicate your chosen consequences one time—and no explanation or rationale is necessary. Once you have communicated the potential consequences, you need to act on them, immediately, in the moment. Otherwise, you lose credibility.
- **Realize that setting boundaries is not a one-time event:** Instead, it is a continual process. Don't expect to set a boundary one time and then be able to stick to it from that time forward. You may have to set a boundary or draw a line in the sand many times before it becomes a natural thing for you to enforce it.
- **Have an exit plan:** Even if you haven't made it clear which behaviors you will no longer accept, *you have a right to exit any unhealthy interaction at any time.* You don't need his permission, and you don't need to warn him. You don't even need to let him know what you are doing. You have a right to take care of yourself in any way that works for you. This is especially true if you have tried telling him how his behavior affects you and have asked him to stop. For example, if your partner is becoming verbally abusive, you can glance at your watch and say, "Oh my gosh, I'm late for an appointment." Or look at your phone and say, "I'm sorry, I have to take this call." It doesn't matter that you are not being completely honest. It is far more important that you take care of yourself.

- **Don't allow yourself to be interrogated:** When your partner asks you a question that you know could end with him criticizing you, don't feel compelled to answer. For example, if he asks you about how much you spent on something and he has a history of criticizing your spending, avoid the potential criticism by merely saying, "Oh, not much." Then bring up something that he likes to talk about—himself.
- **Don't allow yourself to be criticized:** If your partner is extremely critical of you and is constantly finding fault, remember: the less you share of a personal nature, the less information he will have against you. If he criticizes something you are doing, say something like "I feel good about what I did" or "I will keep what you've said in mind." Don't argue, and don't try to convince him that he's wrong about you.
- **Name what is happening:** Some abusers, especially narcissists, test to see what they can get away with. Naming what they are doing will let them know they are not going to get away with it. For example, if he is putting you down, you can say, "That sounded like a put-down." When he talks over you or dismisses what you've said, you can say, "I notice that you don't allow me to finish what I'm saying."

If You Decide to Stay with a Narcissist

If you decide to stay with a partner who is narcissistic, it will be important to understand this disorder as much as possible, not for the purpose of changing him, but so you will better understand how to take care of yourself and how to live in peace with him. There are many books on identifying and living with a narcissist, and I include many in the recommended reading section of the book.

Narcissism has received a lot of attention lately in both psychology and political circles. It is a primary cause of abusive behavior and the core problem of many who suffer from addictions. Despite his air of self-sufficiency, the narcissistic individual is actually more needy than most people. But to admit that he is needy, to admit that a person or a relationship is important to him, forces him to face feelings of deficiency. This, in turn, will create intolerable emptiness, jealousy, and rage inside him. To prevent this from occurring, he must find a way to get his needs met without acknowledging his needs or the person who meets them. This he accomplishes by viewing people as objects or a need-fulfilling function.

The narcissistic individual remains aloof from other people and tends to have only transient social relationships. Because he cannot acknowledge that he needs others, he is almost incapable of feeling true gratitude. Instead, he wards off this feeling by demeaning the gift or the giver. He can be charming when he wishes to impress others and does give the perfunctory "thank you" when it is required socially, but his words are not deeply felt.

With his spouse and family, the narcissistic individual does not even pretend to be grateful. They belong to him and are supposed to meet his every need. Not only will his spouse's and his children's efforts to please him not be appreciated, but they also can always count on his criticism when what is offered is beneath his standards.

The narcissist has no desire to develop his genuine self; he is in love with his false self—the self that wants to deal only with the pleasant, happy, beautiful side of life. This fixation cuts him off from a full range of life experiences and emotional responses. As long as nothing infiltrates his cocoon, he will not be aware of any serious personality problems. He thinks that he has it all and that those who know him will agree since he has carefully selected them to be part of his world and thereby bolster his view of himself.

Despite his aura of grandiosity and his bubble of self-sufficiency, the narcissistic individual is extremely thin-skinned. He constantly takes offense at the way people treat him (e.g., they don't treat him with enough respect, they don't appreciate him enough) and frequently feels mistreated. This may be the only chink in his other-wise thick armor, the only clue that there is something wrong with him. But don't be fooled, the person with NPD is suffering from a serious psychological disorder. While the narcissistic individual may not feel the emptiness in his life, his behavior and attitude cause suffering to all those with whom he has intimate contact.

Typically, those who suffer from NPD or who have strong nar-cissistic traits only seek treatment when they fail to live up to their own expectations of greatness or when their environment fails to support their grand illusions. At this time, they will likely become depressed and seek psychotherapy to ease the pain.

Strategies to Help You Better Communicate and Cope with a Narcissistic Partner

It is very important when dealing with a narcissistic individual or someone with strong narcissistic traits to keep remembering that he is not a very conscious human being, especially when it comes to his own behavior. Although much of his behavior can be experi-enced as emotionally abusive (e.g., his arrogance, his dismissive attitude, his need to be right), he isn't necessarily trying to make you feel bad about yourself. In fact, the primary goal of the nar-cissist is to make himself feel good, even at the expense of others. His inattentiveness, his brashness, and his insensitive comments may seem as if he is deliberately trying to hurt you, but in reality, most of the time he frankly could not care less about how you feel. Most narcissistic individuals are oblivious to others and to the feelings of others. The only time you become important is if you upset the status quo in any of the following ways:

· He needs or wants something from you but isn't getting it.
· You confront him.

- You threaten to change things.
- You threaten to end the relationship.

For this reason, it is important not to take what a narcissistic individual says or does personally. This, of course, is a very difficult task. But if you can try to remember that in a narcissistic individual's world, he is the center of the universe and all the other people are but mere satellites revolving around him, it might help. This doesn't mean he doesn't have feelings or that he isn't capable of caring about others, but it does mean that his needs will always come first.

The only time most narcissistic individuals deliberately try to hurt others is when they themselves feel criticized or threatened in some way (e.g., if you dare to question their ability or knowledge, if you tell them they are wrong about something, or if you challenge their authority). This is when you will feel their full wrath. Narcissistic individuals can cut you to your core in seconds by using just the right words that can wound you the most.

Here are some other suggestions and strategies to help alleviate a great deal of the emotional abuse that can occur in a relationship with a narcissistic person:

- **Recognize that a narcissistic individual has a tremendous need for personal space**. If you insist on too much closeness, he will feel smothered and will lash out at you in order to push you away.
- **Begin to recognize his tendency to criticize.** His criticism can be a sign that he (1) needs some space from you, (2) is feeling critical of himself, or (3) is testing you to see whether you are his equal. Confront him about his criticalness, ask him if he needs more space, and certainly don't buy into his criticalness by asking questions or arguing with him.
- **If he becomes critical of you, call him on it immediately.** The more you allow him to criticize you, the more

he will disrespect you and the more he will continue to criticize you.

· **Don't allow your partner to get a rise out of you.** Narcissists, in particular, love to get a reaction out of people. But showing vulnerability or reacting emotionally (getting upset or arguing with them) increases the risk that they will put you down even more. Of course, because narcissists are masters at getting a rise out of others, it will be difficult to not react, despite your best intentions. When this happens, change the subject or excuse yourself. (Even a bathroom break can help you escape his clutches.)

· **If you have a complaint, state it clearly and strongly.** Don't beat around the bush, don't try to be sensitive and say it subtly. This will only enrage him. And don't whine. Narcissistic individuals hate it when people whine or act like a victim, and they lose all respect for you when you do. When you have a complaint, follow it with a clear statement of how you would like him to change. For example, say something like this: "I don't like the way you dismissed my comment as if it had absolutely no merit. You need to recognize that my opinions are as valid as yours."

· **Refuse to allow yourself to be charmed or used by your partner.** Only do what you really feel like doing, and don't allow yourself to be talked into anything you don't really want to do.

· **Take more responsibility for making sure you get a chance to talk.** Instead of sitting patiently while he goes on and on about himself or his projects, tell him you'd like to share something that happened to you. If he refuses to stop talking, say something like: "I've been listening to you now for quite some time. I'd appreciate it if you'd give me a turn to talk." If this still doesn't work, say something like: "I'm tired of listening to you and not being heard. I'm going to go now."

· **Remember that narcissistic individuals only respect those they feel are their equals.** While they may seek out relationships in which they can feel superior and in which they can control the other person, these people are mere puppets to them. In order for a narcissistic individual to truly care about another person, he must respect her. This means you need to stop putting yourself in a subservient position to him. Start making your own decisions instead of asking for his advice or permission, and start speaking up when he is abusive, insulting, or dismissive.

· **Remind yourself of whom you are dealing with.** Remember: narcissists are people who may act like they are confident and in control, but deep down inside they are needy, empty, and feel inferior. Remembering this will help you feel less intimidated and small around them. It will also help you take their words and their actions less personally and less seriously.

· **Realize that while he can dish out criticism, he can't take it.** This is especially true if it involves "pulling his covers off"—exposing the vulnerabilities and weaknesses under his façade. In fact, even constructive criticism is experienced as a deep wounding in the narcissistic individual. This feeling of being wounded is so profound and so specific to narcissistic individuals that there is a psychological term for it: "narcissistic wounding." When you suggest or point something out to him, don't be surprised if he takes it as a criticism and reacts very strongly. He may lash out at you, he may huff out of the room, or he may give you the silent treatment. You may be able to help the situation by saying to him at a later time, "I didn't mean to hurt your feelings. I was only trying to make a suggestion," or, "I'm sorry if I hurt your feelings. I was only trying to point something out that might help you."

- **Have compassion for yourself.** As you have been learning, self-compassion can help you get through even the most difficult of times. But it can also help you to keep going when things get particularly rough and to not become self-critical if you can't always follow the above suggestions. If you slip and don't enforce your own boundaries, remind yourself that a narcissist's tactics are very powerful and that you have been damaged by years of his abuse. Tell yourself that you are doing the best you can and move on.

The main point to remember is you must stop the narcissistic individual from abusing you. Even though he may not have intended to hurt your feelings, even though he may react very negatively at the time, confronting him is the only way to stop his abusiveness and the only way to gain or retain his respect. If he does make a positive change in his behavior, be sure to acknowledge it. Don't belabor the point, since doing so may cause him to feel too vulnerable and his pride may rise up, causing him to be angry with you. Just acknowledge the change briefly and thank him for making it.

Unfortunately, once a narcissistic individual loses respect for you, it may be nearly impossible to regain it. It depends on how much you've allowed him to control you or abuse you in the past, how much whining and groveling you've done, and how much you've allowed him to see your neediness and vulnerability.

If he shows no signs of respect for you whatsoever—he sighs and rolls his eyes when you talk, he laughs at you when you try to stand up to him, he challenges you to try to live without him—then there is little chance of ever gaining his respect and the relationship will continue to be an abusive one. Your best bet is to work on gaining enough strength to end the relationship. If you choose to stay, all you can do is cut off his aggressiveness and abusiveness by confronting it at the moment and work on building a strong enough sense of self that your partner cannot erode your identity.

Please note: all the above advice on how to cope with a narcissistic person pertains to your regular run-of-the-mill narcissist—not a malignant narcissist. If you are involved with a malignant narcissist, there is no hope for the relationship improving, no matter how carefully you speak with him. If you are involved with a malignant narcissist, you are in danger. Please find a good therapist who specializes in emotional abuse so you can find a way to leave this person.

If You Decide to Stay with a Person Who Has Borderline Personality Disorder

If you decide to stay with a partner who has been diagnosed with BPD or who has strong borderline tendencies, it is important that you learn everything you can about the disorder. Read books on the disorder (see the Recommended Reading list for suggestions) and look online at BPD websites. You also need to recognize that there may be more than one problem occurring. For example, if your partner is male, NPD, substance abuse, and inappropriate use of pornography are common issues that happen simultaneously with BPD.

Accept that if you choose to stay in the relationship, there will be behaviors you will need to learn to tolerate. Those with BPD have distorted thoughts, emotions, and behaviors, as well as behaviors such as splitting (seeing things as black or white, all or nothing), mood swings, intense uncontrollable emotions, feelings of superiority, and suicidal gestures.

One behavior characteristic of those with BPD is intense anger, often referred to as *borderline rage*. Another common characteristic is *impulsive behavior*, which can include physical aggression. While having BPD alone does not suggest a tendency for violence, those with BPD are more likely to suffer from anxiety and substance abuse, which do raise the risk of violence. In addition, those with BPD or who fall somewhere on the borderline spectrum were often victims of violence and may have learned to use aggression to deal with strong emotions. And finally, people with BPD often experience an unstable sense of self and difficulty trusting others in interpersonal relationships. They may experience very strong emotions if they believe they are being rejected or abandoned, and these intense feelings of rejection can sometimes lead to aggressive behaviors.

If your partner has not shown any violent tendencies or aggression, it is quite possible she won't become violent. On the other hand, if you are feeling threatened, even if no violence has occurred in your relationship, you should take those feelings seriously. It is possible the situation could escalate to the point of violence.

Strategies to Help You Better Communicate and Cope with a Partner with Borderline Personality Disorder

Learning to effectively communicate with someone who suffers from BPD or has strong borderline traits can be extremely difficult. Your partner tends to focus most or all of her irrational, intense anger on you, and you likely often feel manipulated, controlled, and lied to. You have probably realized that your partner is either unable or unwilling to admit when she is wrong or has made a mistake. In order to cope with all of these behaviors, you must come to realize that those on the borderline spectrum often experience distortions in their perceptions and therefore cannot be expected to respond to your attempts at logic or rationality.

When dealing with a partner who has BPD:

- **Determine your limits and set appropriate boundaries around what you will accept and what you will not.** Women and men who become involved with a partner who suffers from BPD soon discover that their partner

is a deeply unhappy person. Many learn that their partner had a desperately unhappy childhood, often suffering
from either physical or sexual abuse or severe neglect
and abandonment. Under the circumstances, it is natural
for you to want to be a positive influence in your partner's life and to somehow make up for the severe pain
and loneliness she experienced in the past. Unfortunately,
this may have led you to put up with unacceptable behavior and to swallow your anger and ignore your own
needs. This is what is commonly referred to as codependent behavior on your part. (Codependents typically
avoid their own problems by focusing on those of someone else.) Understand that you are not helping a partner
with BPD by subordinating your own needs and by putting up with unacceptable behavior. In fact, this enables
or reinforces inappropriate behavior on the part of your
partner. With no negative consequences for her actions,
she has no motivation to change.

· **Identify your partner's triggers.** Those who have BPD
or strong borderline tendencies tend to react sponta-
neously and sometimes intensely to certain situations,
words, or actions. These are called triggers. Knowing
what your partner's triggers are can help you avoid
some conflicts. For example, *perceived abandonment* is a
huge trigger for those with BPD, so know ahead of time
that by setting limits you will likely be perceived as shut-
ting her out. Your need for time away from the
relationship will likely be perceived as you pulling away
from her or even as you ending the relationship. Knowing this may help you to anticipate her reaction, be more
sensitive to her feelings when she reacts, and stay detached so you don't get sucked into her drama. When
she reacts strongly to your need for space, you can assure her that you are not abandoning her by saying

something like, "I promise you I will be back," or "I love you, but I just need a break. I'll be back soon." Of course, you cannot avoid all her triggers all the time, and you must keep in mind that your partner's behavior is her responsibility, not yours.

· **Get a reality check.** Those who suffer from BPD or borderline tendencies often suffer from distorted perceptions, especially when it comes to how they view their partner. For example, they often accuse their partner of saying and doing things that he simply did not say or do. For this reason, it is important to get a reality check from time to time. If you become confused as to whether or not you are guilty of the behavior or attitude that your partner is accusing you of, check it out with close friends or family members. While it is not usually advisable for partners in a relationship to involve others in their domestic problems, in your situation it may be the only way you can stay clear as to what is the truth about you and what is a projection or fantasy on your partner's part. Since borderline individuals can also be very perceptive about others and may be the only people who are willing to tell you the truth about yourself, it can be even more confusing. For example, your partner may complain to you that you are insensitive to her needs and too focused on yourself. You may not feel that this is true since you spend a great deal of time trying to make her happy, but after hearing this complaint over and over, you might come to doubt your perceptions. If this is the case, it is time for a reality check. It's quite possible that you are overly self-focused, since it is common for those who suffer from BPD and those with NPD to become involved with one another. But it is also possible that your partner is projecting (attributing her own denied qualities onto you) or confusing you with one of her parents.

Of course, you can't always depend on your friends or family to consistently tell you the truth, but if you let them know it is important and that you would appreciate their honesty, they will likely tell you how they really perceive you. While you might be different with your friends and family than you are with your partner, it's more than likely they have observed you in various situations and with previous lovers and that you can probably trust their perception of you.

· **Remind yourself that you can't always trust your partner's perceptions of you.** If it becomes clear that your partner is projecting her qualities onto you, begin to mirror your partner's projections instead of taking them in. Those who suffer from BPD tend to project their own feelings onto others, particularly their partner. Many partners tend to absorb these projections and soak up their pain and rage. They take much of what their partner says personally and feel that is it their responsibility to make things better. Mason and Kreger, the authors of *Stop Walking on Eggshells*, call this "sponging."

Instead of acting like a sponge, try acting more like a mirror. Reflect your partner's painful feelings back to the rightful owner. Don't get caught up in the accusations, blaming, impossible demands, and criticism. Do this by taking the following steps:

- Maintain your own sense of reality despite what your partner is saying.
- Continue to get reality checks.
- Reflect your partner's projections back to her. For example, if she accuses you of being angry all the time, ask her if she is feeling angry, not in an accusatory way, but coming from a place of curiosity.
- Offer your partner support and understand that she is going through a difficult time.

- Make it clear that while you feel bad that your partner is suffering, she is the only person who can control her feelings and reactions.
- Show by your actions that there are limits to the type of behavior you will accept.
- Communicate these limits and act on them consistently.

· **Learn when to disengage.** If your partner is unable to or refuses to honor the limits you have set or if a situation arises that threatens to get out of hand, the best thing you can do is to emotionally or physically disengage from her. Don't stubbornly continue to assert your point of view when you can see that it is triggering your partner or causing her to become enraged. In her emotional state, she will not be able to really hear you or take in your perspective anyway, and if you persist, she is likely to resort to name-calling, character assassination, or suicidal threats. And don't feel obligated to continue a discussion that has eroded into an argument just because your partner wants to continue it. Here are some suggestions for ways to disengage:

- Change the subject or refuse to continue the discussion.
- Say no firmly and stick to it.
- Leave the room or the house if necessary.
- If the discussion or argument occurs on the phone, hang up and refuse to answer if she calls back.
- Stop the car or refuse to drive until your partner has calmed down.
- If you don't live together, stop seeing your partner for a while.
- Suggest that you continue the discussion in your therapist's office.

There will be times when none of these suggestions work, when your partner has completely lost control. Your suggestion to table the discussion or your attempt to walk away may be interpreted as rejection or abandonment, and your partner may become enraged, attempt to prevent you from leaving, or threaten suicide. In these situations, you should stop trying to handle the situation yourself. If your partner is in therapy, call her therapist. If she is not, call a crisis line. If she threatens violence toward you or herself, call the police.

BPD is a serious personality disorder. Many of those suffering from the disorder don't just threaten suicide, they actually go through with it. And some can become extremely violent if they feel provoked. It is very important that you seek outside help from a competent mental health professional if your attempts at coping with the situation and stopping the emotional abuse seem to upset your partner to the point that she threatens your life or hers.

Make a Distinction Between What You Can Control and What You Cannot

No matter how hard you try, a partner with BPD may not respond as you would like during any particular emotional exchange, discussion, or disagreement. This is beyond your control. What is within your control is how you choose to react to the situation, whether you do all you can to take care of yourself, and whether you do your part in helping to eliminate the emotional abuse in your relationship. This includes working on your own issues.

As mentioned earlier, many partners of those with borderline tendencies or BPD are codependent. There are many definitions of a codependent person, but the one that is most appropriate for your situation is *"a person who avoids his or her own problems and issues by focusing on the problems and issues of his or her partner."* If you are codependent, join Codependents Anonymous (CODA), read books on codependency, or enter therapy to work on your issues. If you have control issues, especially if you have the need to make everyone happy, work to discover the origin of this need so you don't continue taking responsibility for your partner's happiness. There is a strong possibility that you may focus on the needs of others in order to avoid your own unresolved issues. You may feel it is up to you to make others happy because this was the message you received from your parents. Or you may be carrying tremendous guilt or shame, either because you were deeply shamed as a child or because you did something you feel enormous guilt about. If you have low self-esteem, enter therapy to discover the causes and to develop ways to build up your self-confidence and improve your self-image so you will be in a better position to depersonalize and deflect your partner's criticism.

Don't blame all the problems in the relationship on your partner's BPD. For example, if your partner accuses you of something, before writing it off as her typical blaming and criticizing, ask yourself if there is any truth to what she is saying. Those with BPD can be very intuitive, and many of them are extremely sensitive to cues such as body language and tone of voice. Being honest with yourself and owning up to how you are truly feeling will help your partner to trust you and may defuse a potentially explosive situation.

By acknowledging how your behavior may have contributed to the problem, you can act as a healthy role model to your partner. Don't, however, take on more than your share of the responsibility.

It is your choice if you decide to stay with an abusive partner. But you do need to know that there is nearly always a price to pay when you do and that this price may be too high. Think carefully about the potential consequences of your decision, and do everything that is possible to find ways to take care of yourself. Setting healthy boundaries is certainly something to seriously consider. Even so, there are no guarantees that your actions will always have positive outcomes. If you say or do nothing when your partner criticizes, insults, or demeans you, you will likely lose respect for yourself and begin to lose touch with who you really are. On the other hand, if you stand up for yourself, you may incur your partner's wrath. So it is important to know that you may be in a no-win situation.

PART IV

AFTER YOU LEAVE

CHAPTER 13

Fighting the Temptation to Go Back

I wondered about the explorers who'd sailed their ships to the end of the world. How terrified they must have been when they risked falling over the edge: how amazed to discover, instead, places they had seen only in their dreams.
—JODI PICOULT, *Handle with Care*

THOSE WHO ARE FINALLY ABLE to end an abusive relationship often find, much to their dismay, that they are sometimes tempted to go back to their abuser. If this happens to you, remember: this doesn't mean you are weak or masochistic. It just means that it is difficult to let go of someone you love, difficult to leave the past behind, and difficult to start all over again. In this chapter, I address these difficulties head-on and offer step-by-step suggestions for how to deal with them in a way that exhibits self-care and a desire for a better life.

Step One: Seriously question whether you are tempted to go back because you are afraid of being alone, afraid you can't make it on your own, or afraid of the unknown.

You may have only negative associations or memories about being alone. For example, you may have been left alone a lot as a child, and this may have been a frightening experience. Or you may have memories of deep sadness and loneliness because you often had no one to comfort you or keep you company, even in difficult times. You may have associated being alone with feeling unloved, unwanted, or unacceptable. Your thinking may have been: "*There must be something wrong with me, otherwise my parents (and others) would want to be around me.*" For any or all of these reasons, being alone now may catapult you back in time and bring up sad and painful memories. You may feel overwhelmed and desperate, imagining being alone for the rest of your life.

You may also be afraid to be on your own. This is also understandable. It may be the first time in your life you have been completely on your own, especially if you went directly from your parents' home to marriage. The chances are your ex-partner was constantly telling you what to do—even what to think. As much as this made you feel incompetent, his or her controlling ways may have also kept you from having to make your own decisions. Needing to make your own decisions now—about everything from what kind of job to look for to who you can associate with—can be a daunting task. Having to be completely responsible for yourself can feel overwhelming.

You may have spent your entire lifetime feeling like life was controlling you instead of you being in charge of your own life. You may have felt like others were always the ones in charge, always the ones making the rules. If this is the case, it can be particularly challenging for you to be on your own—away from your partner, solely responsible for your own life, no one telling you what to do, needing to make your own decisions and guiding your own path.

It is important that you come to realize that you are fully capable of directing your own path. You don't need anyone telling you what to do or how to be. Your task is to find this out for yourself, and the best way to do this is to step out, to take the risk of individuating, to step away from everyone—your parents, your ex-partner—and declare yourself to the world. Like an artist taking the risk of presenting his or her artwork to the public, you now have the opportunity to present your true self to the world.

You can begin by saying what you really feel instead of what you think you should say, including saying no more often. You can do something you've always wanted to do but were too afraid to take the chance. You can take a class or sign up to go back to school. You can focus on taking care of your mind, body, and spirit better than you ever have before.

It will no doubt be difficult for a while, but instead of running back to your abuser, give yourself a chance to find out that you can make it on your own. In time, you will begin to understand that you have more ability, more strength, and more personal power than you've thought you had. And in time, you can discover that being alone is not the worst thing in the world. Instead of associating being alone with abandonment, rejection, or a sign of your being unwanted or unlovable, it can become associated with freedom and independence.

Step Two: Notice how you feel since you ended the relationship.

Although it will no doubt be painful to be without your partner and you will undoubtedly grieve the ending of the relationship, most people who end an emotionally abusive relationship soon realize that there are some positive things happening with them. Here is a sampling of some of the things former clients have shared with me after a few months or even a few weeks of leaving their abusive partner:

- "I feel a quietness inside of me. It feels strange, but it feels good. I normally have a lot of chatter going on inside my head—critical self-talk, criticisms, and insults from my partner—but now I just notice quiet."
- "I feel at peace with myself. I haven't felt this way in years."

- "I notice I am taking care of myself better."
- "I almost feel bad to say this, but I'm feeling happy."
- "I notice that I'm more often in my body and in the present. I'm not dissociating as much."
- "I absorbed so much of what my partner dumped on me. I believed what he told me without question. Now I'm going back in my mind and realizing that what he said about me wasn't true. I'm seeing myself in a totally different light. I actually like myself now."
- "I have more self-confidence now that I'm away from her. In fact, I'm remembering that I had a lot more self-confidence before I got involved with my wife."
- "I'm not confused all the time."
- "I'm more comfortable in my own skin."
- "I always thought I was the problem in the relationship. Now I can see it was him. He was the problem."
- "I no longer feel hopeless about my life. More and more, I'm feeling more hopeful, more optimistic."
- "I have more energy and enthusiasm than I've had in a long time."
- "I lost myself in my relationship with my husband. Now I'm rediscovering myself. I'm finding my way back to myself."
- "I always focused on his needs, on becoming what he wanted me to be. Now it feels good to focus on myself and my own healing."
- "I notice that even colors seem brighter."

WHAT SEEMS BETTER

Write down all the things that you notice that seem better since you've ended the relationship. This can include things about yourself such as how you are feeling emotionally and physically, the way you perceive yourself, your attitude, the way you operate in the world, and the way you feel around other people. It can also include things about your children, such as that they seem more relaxed, that they are laughing and being silly more often, that they are doing better in school.

As time goes by, you may forget about how different you feel since ending the relationship, so referring to this list can be helpful. It will be especially beneficial to revisit this list when you are going through a particularly difficult time and considering going back. Also, if you end up returning to your partner but discover you made a mistake, having this list available can remind you of how good it felt to be away from him and can give you the courage and strength to leave again.

Step Three: Remember what it was like when you were in the relationship.

Anytime you have the urge to return to your ex-partner, keep in mind the damage the relationship had on your self-esteem, your health, and your sanity, as well as the amount of time it took you to regain your peace of mind. Earlier in the book, I asked you to keep a log of all the abusive incidents you experienced as a way of helping you to face the truth about your situation and to counter periods of denial and "amnesia" as to how bad it really is. I ask that you now go back and retrieve that log and remind yourself of just how bad it got before you ended the relationship. I also encourage you to do the following exercise:

Why I Left

- List all the reasons why you ended the relationship. For example: fear, humiliation, loss of self-esteem, the fact that you had begun to question your perceptions and your very sanity, physical danger, the way the abuse was affecting your children.
- Go over your list from time to time, especially during those times when you feel the strongest pull toward going back to your partner.

Step Four: Weigh the pros and cons of going back to your abuser.

It is understandable that you might miss the positive aspects of your previous life with the abuser and it might just seem easier to go back. Feelings such as these don't necessarily mean you should go back, however. They are just a normal part of the recovery and healing process. The following exercise will help you see the situation in a more realistic way. Take your time and really think about your answers. Be as honest with yourself as you can be.

Balancing the Good and the Bad

1. Make a list of all the reasons why you are considering going back to your partner. For example: financial security, having an intimate partner, having good sex, having the children's father present on a day-to-day basis.

2. Now read over your previous list of all the humiliating, frightening, painful, and traumatic events
   you experienced during your time with the abuser.
   Remember all the times he humiliated you in front
   of others, his constant criticism, his gaslighting, any
   incidents of physical abuse.

3. Ask yourself, "Are the positive things I will gain by
   going back worth the likely negative consequences?"

4. List what you consider to be the positive traits of
   your ex-partner or the positive things he brought
   to the relationship. For example: his sexual attraction toward you, his ability to make a good living,
   the extent to which he loves your children.

5. Now list the negative traits of your ex-partner. Try
   to focus on the characteristics that were damaging
   to you then and would probably be harmful to you
   again if you went back. For example: his controlling
   nature, his shaming statements, his constant criticism, his irrational jealousy.

6. Now compare these two lists and carefully consider
   whether his good qualities outweigh the negative.

If you continue to struggle, you may need to review these
lists more than once. I also recommend counseling at this
point if you haven't already started.

Step Five: Consider whether your ex-partner has made any significant
changes.

Most abusers suffer from chronic shame, and they need to heal
this shame if they are going to be able to stop being abusive. In
order to address chronic shame, the abuser must engage in ongoing,

intensive psychotherapy. This form of therapy includes developing a meaningful relationship with a therapist, and this means the abuser needs to develop enough trust in the therapy and the process to let down his defensive wall and become vulnerable enough to show his true self to the therapist and to himself. Unless your ex-partner engages in this type of therapy with a professional who has worked successfully with abusers, there is little to no hope for real, lasting change. This means that even if you observe some changes today, these changes will not likely last on a long-term basis. They are behavioral changes rather than changes that come from the abuser's deep understanding of himself. In addition, most abusers need empathy training since many lack this important ability.

The Changes the Abuser Needs to Make

There are specific changes your ex-partner needs to make in order to no longer be a threat to you. These include:

1. **He needs to be able to admit to you that he was emotionally abusive toward you and/or your children.** He also needs be able to state clearly *how* he was abusive (specifically what forms of abuse he was guilty of). He needs to be consistent about this—no backtracking, minimizing, discrediting your memory, or blaming you.
2. **He needs to exhibit empathy toward you and others he harmed.** This means he needs to show that he has been able to put himself in your place and has begun to truly understand how you felt when he acted in abusive ways.
3. **He needs to understand and to acknowledge to you how his abusiveness harmed you and/or your children.** He needs to be able to name in detail the short and long-term effects that his abuse has had on you and your children, including fear, shame, loss of self-

confidence, loss of trust, loss of important relationships, and loss of freedom.

4. **He needs to be able to do the above steps without feeling sorry for himself or talking about how hard the experience has been for *him*.**

5. **If she has a personality disorder such as BPD or NPD, she needs to admit this to herself and to you and seek professional help.** Specifically, she needs to come to realize how her disorder caused her to be emotionally abusive, even if she didn't intend to do so.

6. **He needs to accept the consequences of his actions, including you leaving him.** This means he has to stop blaming you or whining about his losses or the problems he has experienced as the result of his abuse (e.g., loss of the marriage, your loss of desire to have sex with him, money problems).

7. **He needs to make amends for the damage he has done.** This includes giving you a *meaningful apology*. (Please refer back to chapter 10 for details on what composes a meaningful apology.)

8. **He needs to be able to understand and talk about the underlying beliefs and values that drove his abusive behaviors.** These include viewing himself as superior to others, considering himself entitled to constant attention or special treatment, or believing that women can't be trusted.

9. **He needs to have developed respectful behaviors and attitudes to replace his past abusive ones.** You should be able to notice such things as him listening to you more, not always having to be right, not blaming you every time something goes wrong in his life, not becoming possessive and jealous when you venture out in the world or make new friends, and carrying his weight in household chores and childcare.

10. **She needs to have replaced her distorted image of you with a more accurate picture of who you are.** That is, she needs to recognize your strengths, abilities, and achievements.

11. **He needs to commit to not repeating his abusive behaviors.** This needs to be without conditions such as promising to stop calling you names as long as you respect him. He needs to back up his words of commitment by seeking counseling or entering into a treatment program.

12. **He needs to accept that overcoming abusiveness will be a lifetime process.** He can't announce that he is cured and that therefore you should take him back.

13. **He needs to stop pressuring you to go back or to make a decision.** This in itself can become abusive. If you need time to decide whether to go back or not, he should be able to give you that time—without threatening you, without trying to make you feel guilty.

Some of the items above are adapted from a list in Lundy Bancroft's book *Why Does He Do That? Inside the Minds of Angry and Controlling Men*. Although his book was written about physically abusive men, much of it applies to emotional abuse as well. I suggest you read his book to get a better understanding of the dynamics of an abuser.

Step Six: Begin the process of grieving your ex-partner.

A divorce or the ending of an intimate relationship represents the death of that relationship and all the hopes and dreams that went into it. And the death of a relationship, like any death, requires a grieving process to take place in order for healing to occur.

Oftentimes, former victims are afraid of going through the grieving process. They are afraid that once they allow themselves to begin to grieve their partner and/or the relationship, they won't be able to tolerate the pain. Going back to their partner may seem to be the lesser of two evils. For this reason, it can help to understand the process of grief.

Grief is a natural response to loss. It affects the body, mind, and spirit. Symptoms can include extreme sadness, loss of appetite, insomnia, disorientation, inability to focus, hopelessness, suicidal thoughts, lack of motivation, forgetfulness, anger, anxiety, and depression.

There are very good reasons why we resist feeling and expressing our emotions of sadness and grief when a relationship ends, including:

- Fear that if you begin to cry you will never stop
- Fear that you will become deeply depressed if you allow yourself to feel your pain
- Fear that you don't have the emotional strength to endure the pain
- Fear that allowing yourself to grieve will transport you back in time and that you will be unable to come back to the present

Let's examine these fears one by one.

- **The fear that if you begin to cry you will never stop.** I remember what a very wise therapist once told me when I asked her, "How long am I going to cry like this?" She said, "You will cry until you have no more tears to cry." Although it can be scary when you end up crying for a long time, the good news is that your body will take care of you. Your sobs may cause you to cough and even choke momentarily at times, but your body will not allow you to cry to the point where you are endangering yourself. You will either become short of breath and will need

to stop to catch your breath or you will become so exhausted that you fall asleep.

· **The fear of becoming so overwhelmed with grief that
you become depressed.** This is a very understandable
fear. The truth is, you are more likely to become depressed if you do *not* allow yourself to express your pain
and grief. Nevertheless, we don't want you to get stuck
in your sadness and grief so much that you can no longer
experience any good in the world. I am going to teach
you techniques that will help you to feel your deep sadness without becoming overwhelmed by it. (Of course, if
you feel you are getting stuck in your sadness or grief,
please consult a psychotherapist or medical doctor.)

· **The fear that you do not have the emotional strength to
endure the pain.** You know yourself better than anyone
else. You know how fragile you are at any given time. You
may not feel strong enough at this moment to face your
pain and grieve for your relationship, and that is okay. On
the other hand, you may be a lot stronger than you think.
You may only need to consider what you have already survived to be reminded of just how strong you actually are.
It has taken enormous strength to endure the emotional
pain of the abuse. If you have been crying throughout this
book, your body is telling you that you are sad and that
you need to let out the tears. Let them start flowing.

· **The fear that you will get stuck in the past.** While this
is a valid fear, I will offer you ways of grounding yourself
in the present so that you don't stay stuck in your past
feelings or in your past traumas.

There are techniques and strategies that you can use to protect yourself so that your worst fears don't come true. These
include new ways to confront and process your pain over having
been abused and ways to allow yourself to grieve your losses. I
am confident that you can engage in these processes without

being further traumatized. If, however, you feel too overwhelmed or traumatized, I recommend you seek professional help if you haven't already done so.

The following two exercises will help you to remain grounded and in the present while you grieve.

BASIC GROUNDING EXERCISE

1. Find a quiet place where you will not be disturbed or distracted.
2. Sit up in a chair or on a couch. Put your feet flat on the ground. If you are wearing shoes with heels, you will need to take your shoes off so that you can have your feet flat on the ground. Now pay attention to where your feet touch the ground. Feel that connection.
3. With your eyes open, take a few deep breaths. Turn your attention once again to feeling the ground under your feet. Continue your breathing and feeling your feet flat on the ground throughout the exercise.
4. Now, as you continue breathing, take a look around the room. Notice the colors, shapes, and textures of the objects around you.
5. Bring your focus back to feeling the ground under your feet as you continue to breathe, but also continue to notice the different colors, textures, and shapes of the objects in the room.

This grounding exercise will serve several purposes:

· It will bring your awareness back to your body, which in turn can stop you from being triggered or from dissociating.

- It will bring you back to the present, to the here and now—a good thing if you have been triggered and have been catapulted back into the past.
- Deliberately focusing your attention outside yourself by being visually involved in the world breaks the shame spiral and allows those feelings and thoughts to subside.
- It will help you to focus on being mindful.

I recommend you also use this grounding technique whenever you find yourself triggered by a past memory or when you find yourself "leaving your body" or dissociating, which is common for trauma victims.

THE WAVE

The following steps will help you to experience your emotions as you grieve without becoming overwhelmed by them. You can also practice this exercise anytime you feel an intense emotion, whether it is pain, fear, anger, or shame.

1. Prepare for this exercise by grounding yourself.
2. Begin by simply observing your emotion. Notice how it makes you feel. Notice what happens in your body as you feel the emotion. Do not judge the emotion as good or bad.
3. Fully experience your emotion. Allow yourself to feel the emotion as a wave, coming and going. Try not to suppress the feelings or push the emotion away. On the other hand, don't hold on to the emotion or amplify it. Just let it rise up like a wave and then subside.

4. Step back from your emotion. This experience of simply "witnessing" an emotion will put you in a better position to detach from it and to let go of the intense energy you may have invested in it.

5. Get unstuck from the emotion. Once you are more detached from the emotion, you can begin to let it go: it has served its purpose.

The previous two exercises will help you when you are suddenly overwhelmed with grief as well as when you deliberately set aside time to grieve. The following exercise will help prevent you from suddenly being triggered (reminded of your partner) out of the blue.

RE-TRIGGERING EXERCISE

Create a list of dates, occasions, places, and events that remind you of your ex-partner and/or your relationship, things that are likely to trigger painful feelings (birthdays, anniversaries, times of the year). Also note what sounds, smells, music, and movies tend to trigger memories. If at all possible, try to anticipate these triggers and, when you can, avoid these circumstances. For example, you might want to keep the radio in your car turned off after you leave your ex-partner. It is likely that songs that remind you of him will come on. Instead, listen to music that you have chosen on your phone or a CD player that won't trigger memories. On the other hand, if you are having difficulty allowing yourself to cry, you may want to deliberately listen to songs that remind you of your ex-partner.

The Goodbye Letter

This exercise may help you find the best way for you to say goodbye to your ex-partner in a way that is not completely overwhelming.

1. Begin to compose a "goodbye letter" to your ex-partner. Imagine that this will be the last time you get a chance to say what you need to say—to express your anger or to let him or her know how much he or she hurt you.

2. It may take you several sittings before you can complete the letter, so take your time. Your letter may include a lot of anger, or it may be more of an expression of the sadness you feel that the relationship didn't work.

3. Don't be afraid of expressing your loving feelings, but remember that the purpose of the letter is for you to say goodbye.

4. After you have completed your letter, read it through several times, including reading it out loud. This will help you decide whether you want to actually give the letter to your ex-partner.

The Box and the Fire

I designed this exercise to enable you to not "throw the baby out with the bathwater"—to help you keep the good memories and get rid of the bad.

1. Make a copy of the list you previously wrote describing your ex-partner's good qualities or create a new list.

2. Do the same for the list of his negative qualities.

3. Fold the first list up in order to fit it into a box of your choosing. Put this box in a hidden, out-of-the-way place and promise yourself not to open this box for six months. Tell yourself, "I'll let myself remember the good times when I have allowed myself to let go of him—when it is safe to remember the good."

4. Burn the second list, the list of his bad qualities. You can do this by putting the list in the fireplace or a barbeque, or by simply placing the list over a large flat bowl and taking a match to it. As the list burns, tell yourself, "I'm getting rid of all the negativity connected to my ex-partner. I am saying goodbye to the abuse, the pain, the shame, and the fear."

"BURYING" YOUR EX-PARTNER

This last exercise is only recommended to those of you who feel strong enough to complete it, those who are determined to end the relationship once and for all instead of getting sucked back into it. This is what one client who completed this exercise told me: "I needed to get my ex-partner out of my life completely. Even though there was absolutely no reason for me to ever see him again [she had no children with him, and she had moved to another town], I was still haunted by him. It was like he was a permanent presence in my head. I needed to get him out of my consciousness. I needed to exorcise him."

1. Imagine that your ex-partner died and that you need to say goodbye to him. You may even want to go to a cemetery and find a gravesite that can fill in for an imaginary gravesite for your partner.
2. Say goodbye either out loud or inside your head. You can either use the goodbye letter that you have written or you can write a eulogy or another piece of writing that will serve the purpose of you burying and saying goodbye to your ex-partner for good.

Step Seven: Continue to heal from the abuse

This is actually the most important step. Healing takes time and work, and unless you put in this time and work, you are far more likely to either run back to your abuser or to choose another abuser.

Establishing a New Relationship with Your Feelings

Taking a fresh look at difficult emotions like pain, anger, and fear can provide you with important information about what's happening inside of you. Emotions become destructive—meaning that they cause us greater mental or physical suffering—when we either cling to them or push them away. And emotions seem to get stronger the more we fight them. The healthier way to deal with these difficult emotions is to "hold" them in an open, aware, self-compassionate way. You can also change your relationship to your feelings by not judging an emotion or getting upset because you are feeling an emotion. Instead of telling yourself things like "I hate feeling like this" or "I shouldn't feel like this" or "I'm wrong to have this feeling," work toward accepting the emotion with self-compassionate statements like:

- "It is understandable that I would feel sad right now"
- "I have a right to feel angry."

Healing Your Post-Traumatic Stress Disorder

Peter Levine, the author of *Waking the Tiger: Healing Trauma*, has studied stress and trauma for thirty-five years. He has found that when a situation is perceived to be life threatening, as is often the case with intimate partner violence, both our mind and our body mobilize a vast amount of energy in preparation to fight or escape, often referred to as the fight-or-flight response. This is the same energy that can enable a mother to lift a car off her son's legs when he is trapped underneath it. This kind of strength is created by a large increase in the amount of blood to the muscles and the release of stress hormones, such as cortisol and adrenaline.

In the act of lifting the two-thousand-pound car, the mother discharges most of the excess chemicals and energy she has mobilized in order to deal with the threat to her child. This discharge of energy from the body, when complete, informs the brain that the threat is over and that it is time to reduce the levels of stress hormones in the body.

However, if the chemicals and energy are not released and the message to normalize is not given, the brain just continues to release high levels of adrenaline and cortisol and the body remains in a high-energy, ramped-up state. Unlike his mother, this is the situation the son faces. Unless he can find a way to discharge the excess energy brought on by the crisis, his body will continue responding as it did when he was helpless and his body was in pain. This is essentially what happens with those who suffer from PTSD. They experience intense anxiety; have heightened reactions; are easily triggered; experience disturbing thoughts, feelings, dreams, and memories related to the trauma; and avoid situations that bring back memories.

Unfortunately, human beings don't know how to "blow off the stress" of a near-death experience the way animals do. For example, a captured bear that has been shot with a tranquilizer dart will come out of its state of shock once the tranquilizer wears off. It does this by beginning to tremble—lightly at first and then at a steadily intensifying level until it peaks into a near-convulsive shaking, its limbs flailing seemingly at random. After the shaking stops, the animal takes deep, organic breaths that spread throughout its body.

What is even more interesting is that when the bear's response is viewed in slow motion, it becomes obvious that the seemingly random gyrations it is doing during this process are actually coordinated running movements. It is as if the bear is completing its escape by actively finishing the running movements that were interrupted when it was tranquilized by the dart. Then the bear shakes off the "frozen energy" as it surrenders in spontaneous, full-body breaths.

Researchers like Levine explain that people do, in fact, possess the same built-in ability to shake off trauma the way animals do, but that many of us have simply forgotten how to use it. Given the appropriate guidance, human beings can and do shake off the effects of overwhelming events like emotional and physical abuse using exactly the same procedures that animals use.

Levine says that the reason his program, called *somatic therapy*, works is that trauma is primarily physiological. Trauma happens initially to our bodies and our instincts. Only afterward do its effects spread to our minds, emotions, and spirits.

It is important that victims of abuse release the frozen energy trapped in their bodies after an attack—whether it is emotional or physical. If your partner emotionally attacked you, you may have tried to defend yourself or you may have tried to escape. But even so, the damage was done. Now you likely have that unspent rage and fear trapped in your body. Discharging this energy informs the brain that it is time to reduce the levels of stress hormones in the body—that the threat is no longer present. Until the message to normalize is given, the brain just continues to release high levels of adrenaline and cortisol, the body holds on to its high-energy state, *and you continue to feel pain and helplessness.*

Releasing your anger in any of the following ways can help you shake off the stress associated with a physical or emotional attack. Please note: doing any of these exercises can act as a trigger, catapulting you back to the trauma of the attack. This is okay if you are imagining pushing, shoving, or kicking your attacker away and feeling empowered, but if you slip into feeling fear and helplessness, ground yourself (refer to the basic grounding exercise earlier in the chapter) and bring yourself back to the present. Keep doing the exercise until you are completely back in the present.

Stomp It Out

Lie flat on your back on your bed, bend your knees, and place your feet flat on the bed. Now stomp your feet as hard as you can. You can also do this exercise by keeping your legs straight and alternating lifting each leg up and slamming it down hard on the bed. Say "No!" as you do this.

Push It Away

Stand in front of a sturdy door in your house. Put both arms out and place your palms flat against the door. As you push against the door as hard as you can, say "Get away!" or "Get out of here!"

· Many former victims of trauma, including emotional abuse, hold their breath and their bodies tightly, bracing themselves for the next attack. This hypervigilance can take its toll on the body. Creating environments where you can practice deep breathing and relax your body can lower your defenses, helping to heal not only the mind but the body as well. Yoga is a great way to do this. If you can afford it, I also recommend any of the following types of therapies to help you heal your PTSD symptoms: eye movement desensitization and reprocessing therapy (EMDR), cranial-sacral therapy, and Levine's form of therapy called somatic therapy.

THE TRUTH IS, you may still go back to your ex-partner even after focusing on the suggestions I have offered in this chapter. This does not mean you are a failure or that you are a lost cause. In fact, it is common for abuse victims to return to their abuser. You may need to go back because of financial problems or because you truly believe he or she has changed and you feel like he or she deserves another chance. Please don't judge yourself for going back, no matter what the reason. It may actually be better this time or you may discover that it is not. Either way, you did what you felt you had to do.

Going back does not have to end your work on yourself, however. I encourage you to continue reading the book and to continue to heal from your previous abuse experiences. This will make you stronger no matter what happens between you and your ex-partner in the future.

CHAPTER 14

Forgive Yourself by Understanding Yourself

Once you've accepted your flaws, no one can use them against you.

—ANONYMOUS

SHAME IS A PERSISTENT EMOTION. It can hang on long after you have escaped an emotionally abusive relationship. Every time you make a mistake, have a bad day, or experience a setback of some kind, your ex-partner's words can come rising up like a monster from the depths. Even when you find ways to quiet those critical, shaming messages, you may find that you still experience horrible shame when you realize the harm your children have endured or when you think about how long you put up with such abusive behavior.

Instead of continually shaming yourself, you need to forgive yourself. Otherwise you will carry your shame with you indefinitely, making it harder to start your life anew. You need to forgive yourself for all the following: for not seeing the signs and predictors of abusive behavior, for believing what the abuser told you, for getting confused about who you really are, and for continuing the relationship for so long. You may also need to forgive yourself for subjecting your children to the chaos and fighting and for providing them negative role models for how to behave in intimate relationships. Next, you need to forgive yourself for the ways you have hurt others as a result of the abuse you suffered. This includes all the ways you have caused others damage. And finally, you need to forgive yourself for whatever actions you took or coping mechanisms you used in order to survive. In this chapter, I will guide you step-by-step through the process of completing each of these tasks.

Self-forgiveness is an important aspect of self-compassion and is one of the most powerful steps you can take to rid yourself of your debilitating shame. It is not only recommended but absolutely essential: nothing is as important for your overall healing from the abuse. It goes like this: the more shame you heal, the more you will be able to see yourself more clearly instead of through the distorted lens of your abusive ex-partner. Instead of viewing yourself as weak or stupid or incompetent, you will be able to view yourself more realistically and realize that you, like everyone else, can make mistakes, can be imperfect, and that you still deserve to be treated with respect and consideration.

While self-compassion is the antidote to shame, the healing medicine is self-forgiveness. Self-compassion acts to neutralize the poison of shame, to remove the toxins created by shame. Self-forgiveness acts to soothe our body, mind, and soul of the pain caused by shame and facilitates the overall healing process.

Self-Understanding

One of the main tools we will use to help you forgive yourself is *self-understanding*. This includes learning how shame has shaped your image of yourself, how the emotional abuse you suffered cut you off from important aspects of yourself, and how trauma creates certain symptoms and behaviors that are unhealthy.

A major way to gain self-understanding is to begin to use what is called a "trauma-sensitive" or "trauma-informed" approach with yourself. This perspective frames many behaviors as *understandable* attempts to *cope with* or *adapt to* overwhelming circumstances (such as emotional abuse), and it is therefore both empathetic and potentially empowering.

The primary goal of a trauma-sensitive or trauma-informed way of thinking is to help you gain a better understanding of the role that trauma has played in *shaping your life*. More specifically, there is a focus on helping you recognize that many of the behaviors you are most critical of in yourself (and are criticized for by others) are actually *coping mechanisms* or *attempts at self-regulation*. By using this approach, you will not only gain understanding as to why you have behaved as you have but you also will increase your ability to treat yourself in a more compassionate way.

Below are some of the principles of a trauma-informed way of thinking. I encourage you to adopt these principles and beliefs as you continue to focus on healing your shame (as well as other effects of the abuse you suffered).

- The impact of trauma narrows a victim's choices, undermines self-esteem, takes away control, and creates a sense of hopelessness and helplessness.
- Troubling behaviors need to be viewed as attempts to cope with past trauma and seen as *adaptations* rather than *pathologies*.
- It is understood that every behavior helped a victim in the past and continues to help in the present in some way.
- There is a focus on what happened to the person rather than what is wrong with the person.
- Substance use and certain psychiatric symptoms such as self-harm may have evolved as coping strategies at a time when options were limited.
- Victims are doing the best they can at any given time to cope with the life-altering and frequently shattering effects of trauma.

Instead of blaming yourself for your efforts to manage the trauma of emotional abuse, realize that a victim of emotional abuse is likely to react to the trauma by behaving in problematic ways, including abusing alcohol or drugs, other addictions such as gambling and shoplifting, self-harm, or abusive behavior toward their loved ones. Begin to recognize the adaptive function of your behaviors. For example, drinking and other forms of substance abuse often arise out of a victim's efforts to cope with high levels of anxiety—anxiety that can sometimes be intolerable. Recognizing this and having compassion for yourself will be a significant step toward both self-acceptance and change. Once you have offered yourself self-compassion, you can then focus on learning strategies that help you feel more comforted and in control, such as writing in a journal, taking a warm bath, applying a cool washcloth to your forehead, or practicing grounding exercises or deep breathing—all of which can help with self-soothing. (We'll discuss this further in the next chapter.)

Self-understanding can also help you realize why you ended up in an abusive relationship in the first place, as well as why you stayed in one. For example, while any man or woman can find himself or herself in an abusive relationship, there are certain circumstances that can set a person up to enter such a relationship and to have a difficult time leaving an abusive partner. In particular, it has been found that victims of abuse have a history of the following:

- Being emotionally, physically, or sexually abused in childhood
- Being neglected in childhood
- Being emotionally or physically abandoned as a child
- Having a personality disordered parent (narcissist or borderline)
- Having a parent who is an alcoholic or an alcohol or drug abuser

If your childhood history includes any of the above, it is *understandable* that you would have been attracted to an emotionally abusive partner. We will discuss this in more detail later on in the chapter.

By viewing yourself in a trauma-sensitive way, you will become far less critical of yourself, no longer seeing yourself as a "bad person" because you sometimes reacted to the trauma of emotional abuse in troubling ways. And as you come to recognize that the negative things you have done do not represent who you are at your core but are the ways that you learned to cope with the trauma you experienced, my hope is that this self-understanding will help you to forgive yourself and begin to treat yourself in far more compassionate ways.

Starting with the premise that no one is perfect and that we all make mistakes, self-understanding encourages us to view ourselves from the perspective that there is always a reason why we do the things we do. For example, if you are impatient with your children, ask yourself, "Why do I treat my children this way? Does it have anything to do with the way my husband treats me? Have I grown so afraid of being judged and criticized that this fear has trickled down to my children? Am I so afraid that I or they will be criticized that I try to encourage them to be perfect?"

Or could it be that one or both of your parents were impatient with you and that you are passing this behavior down to your children? Did you become impatient and critical of yourself and then pass this tendency down to the way you interact with your children?

If either of these scenarios is true for you, then it is *understandable* that you would become impatient with your children. Understanding why you act as you do is not the same as *excusing* your behavior. It is merely choosing to come from a place of self-understanding rather than a place of criticism. It is the difference between seeing yourself as *bad* for being imperfect and seeing yourself as *human*.

It is *understandable* that if we are treated with impatience, criticism, harshness, and a lack of acceptance, we will treat others—especially our children—the same way. We aren't saints. When we are treated poorly, it affects us deeply, it changes our basic personality structure. As the saying goes, "Hurt people, hurt people." Once you understand yourself and your actions, you can begin to work on self-forgiveness.

The Obstacles to Self-Forgiveness

Just as you probably had a lot of resistance to self-compassion, you also may resist the idea of self-forgiveness. You may view self-forgiveness as "letting myself off the hook." But this is not what we are talking about. We are talking about taking responsibility for your actions but not continuing your relentless self-criticism. Beating yourself up for getting into an abusive relationship or for the ways you coped with it isn't going to help anyone, including yourself. And it certainly won't help you to move forward.

The more shame you feel about your past actions and behaviors, the more your self-esteem is lowered and the less likely it is you will feel motivated to change. And without self-forgiveness, your level of shame will cause you to refuse to see your faults and not be open to criticism or correction. Self-forgiveness opens the door to change by releasing resistance and deepening your connection to yourself.

You may also ask, "Why should I forgive myself? After all, it won't help those I've harmed." The most powerful reason is this: if you do not forgive yourself, the shame you carry will compel you to continue to act in harmful ways toward others and yourself. Forgiving yourself will help you to heal another layer of shame and free you to continue becoming a better human being. Without the burden of self-hatred you have been carrying around, you can literally transform your life.

Forgiving Yourself for the Abuse Itself

Forgiving yourself for the abuse is the obvious place to start. You no doubt felt imprisoned by your abusive partner, but by forgiving yourself for the abuse, you will stop making yourself a prisoner of your own making. As Judith Viorst, the author of the wonderful book *Necessary Losses*, stated, "You may be sentencing yourself to a lifetime of penance for a crime you didn't commit." As I've mentioned many times, victims tend to blame themselves for the abuse because it is preferable to feeling vulnerable and out of control. If you continue to blame yourself for the abuse, you can continue to hold on to the illusion of control and avoid the feelings of helplessness that accompanied the abuse. And equally important, if you can continue to blame yourself for what your abuser did, you don't have to face the feelings of abandonment, betrayal, and disappointment that go hand in hand with facing the truth about someone you cared about.

Hopefully, much of the information offered in the book thus far has helped many of you to stop blaming yourselves for the abuse. But for some people, no matter how many times they hear that they are not to blame for the abuse, they simply do not believe it. They are convinced that they are somehow responsible for the abuse occurring.

Getting Past Your Denial

The first thing you need to do on your path to self-forgiveness is to get past your denial. The primary reason why those who were emotionally abused tend to continue to blame themselves for the abuse is *denial*. Denial is a powerful defense mechanism intended to protect us from having to face intense pain and trauma. It is what allows us to block out or "forget" the intense pain caused by severe physical and emotional trauma. Victims of emotional abuse tend to deny what happened to them and minimize the damage it caused them because to admit to what happened is to face the sometimes unbearable pain that someone they loved could have treated them in such horrendous ways.

One way to help you face the truth once and for all that you were not to blame for the emotional abuse you suffered is to learn more about the traits that are common to people who become abusive. Those who become abusive tend to have certain predictable traits, attitudes, and behavior patterns. If you find that your ex-partner has many or all of the characteristics on the following list, it may help you come out of denial about who the responsible party actually is.

Those who become abusive often have:

- A childhood background involving emotional, physical, or sexual abuse, and/or abandonment issues
- A tendency to blame others for their problems
- A strong desire to remain in control, a fear of being out of control, and/or a need for power and control
- Difficulty empathizing with others or an inability to empathize with others
- An inability to respect interpersonal boundaries, a compulsion to violate boundaries
- A tendency to be unreasonable or to have unreasonable expectations of their children, a partner, and a relationship
- Repressed anger
- An uncontrollable temper (very short fuse and tendency to get angry immediately)
- A tendency to be emotionally needy or demanding, a dependent personality
- Poor impulse control
- Intense fear of abandonment
- High levels of stress and high arousal levels
- Poor coping skills
- Selfishness and narcissism

- A history of being abusive (physically, verbally, and sexually) as an adult or an older child

It is important to understand who abusers are and why they act as they do in order to help you to recognize that *you didn't cause the abuser in your life to become abusive*. An abuser was already abusive before he or she met you. The fact is, *you didn't have to do anything at all to cause this person to become abusive*. He or she didn't emotionally abuse you because you couldn't do anything right, because you were stubborn, because you didn't listen. He or she abused you because it was inevitable due to his or her emotional makeup and background. In other words, this person was a ticking time bomb, just waiting to go off. You just happened to be in the vicinity when he or she did.

Beliefs That Predispose Someone to Becoming Abusive

In addition to a person's background and his or her personality characteristics, those who become emotionally abusive tend to have certain beliefs about themselves and others that set them up to become abusive. These beliefs set the tone for the relationship and can be abusive in themselves. People who become abusers believe that:

- They are always right.
- It is always someone else's fault.
- Their needs are more important than those of others.
- They have a right to expect others to do as they demand, and if someone refuses, he or she is now the enemy.
- They are superior or otherwise "better than" (e.g., smarter, more competent, more powerful) than most people and that therefore they *deserve* special treatment or consideration.

- It is not important what others are feeling.
- Those who complain about their behavior are just too sensitive or too demanding.
- They cannot trust anyone, and others are constantly out to get them.

Again, if your ex-partner had many of the above beliefs, this person has an *abusive personality*. This means that this person is abusive in most of his or her relationships, especially when he or she has all the power.

All of the above information is intended to help you recognize that there is only one person responsible for abusing you—the person doing the abusing. It is never the fault of the person being abused. *Stop blaming yourself for the abuse—it was not your fault, no matter what the circumstances.*

Forgiving Yourself for Choosing an Abusive Partner

I want to make something very clear. There are plenty of victims of abuse who came from healthy families. But there are also many who came from dysfunctional or abusive families in which they had at least one parent who was abusive to his or her partner and/or children. If this is your situation, part of forgiving yourself for the abuse is to come to understand that you were, in fact, *repeating a pattern*. This was the case with my client Kara.

> I don't know why I didn't see it before, but my husband is very much like my abusive father. They have so many of the same characteristics. They are both self-involved and have very little awareness or concern for the feelings of others. On the other hand, they are both extremely thin-skinned and get their feelings hurt all the time. Just as my father constantly complained to

my mother that she didn't care about him, my husband complained about the same thing. He always felt slighted by me. If I wasn't paying constant attention to him, he felt neglected. Now, when I look back, I remember that my father was the same way. Meeting his needs was supposed to be my mother's main job. He expected her to drop whatever she was doing as soon as he came home. My husband had the same expectation. He even called me several times a day to tell me to run errands for him. It was as if he thought my entire existence was to take care of his needs.

Now that I see the similarities between my husband and my father, I realize I was just doing what both my parents taught me to do. To my parents, the woman is supposed to be subservient to the man. My father acted this out in front of us kids all the time, and my mother went along with it and didn't complain. No wonder I married who I did, and no wonder I ended up acting just like my mother!

This new awareness was the key to Kara being able to forgive herself for marrying an abusive man. As soon as she was able to connect her past with her present, she was able to forgive herself for choosing an abusive partner.

My client Randall also discovered he was repeating a pattern by marrying a woman just like his mother. Randall's mother behaved in very erratic, abusive ways when he was growing up. He and his father never knew when something was going to upset her, and so they were always extremely careful around her. His father gave in to any request from his mother, even if it seemed petty or selfish. There were many times when his father would go out late at night, even in bad weather, to bring his mother some kind of food that she was craving. And Randall witnessed his mother constantly accusing his father of something: not caring about her, flirting with other women, or disrespecting her in some way. His father tried to defend himself but to no avail. As far as his mother was concerned, his father was always wrong and had to make amends in some way.

Randall ended up marrying a woman who had the same emotional problems as his mother. Like Randall's mother, his wife exhibited many borderline tendencies—behaviors that ended up being emotionally abusive, even though it was not her intention to be that way. And like his mother, Randall's wife was often irrational, getting upset about the smallest things and magnifying them into huge sins. If Randall was late coming home, she accused him of having an affair or of not wanting to come home. If he looked at her in a certain way, she accused him of being angry with her. Even though the complaints and accusations seemed endless, Randall, like his father, always worked hard to be calm and to try to explain to her that she was misinterpreting his actions.

Another man with a different family background would have probably ended the marriage a long time before Randall was able to do so. That other person would have realized that he was in a no-win situation. Randall, on the other hand, was determined to convince his wife that he loved her, no matter what it took.

This desire to achieve a different outcome despite all the odds is the hallmark of what is called the *repetition compulsion*. This is another way that coming from an abusive or otherwise dysfunctional family can set you up to be attracted to an abusive partner. In an attempt to undo the past and reach a different outcome, many people find that they are intensely attracted to a partner who is a replica of an abusive parent. On an unconscious level, it is as if they believe that if they can get their partner to appreciate them, love them, or not abandon them, it can undo what their abusive parent did to them.

We can be involved in the repetition compulsion even when we deliberately try to find a partner who is different from an abusive or neglectful parent. This was the situation with my client

Kelly, who didn't realize that she had married a man who was a replica of her father. "I just never saw the similarities. In fact, I thought I was marrying a man who was the opposite of my father," she explained during one of her sessions.

Kelly had made the mistake of focusing on outward appearances when choosing a partner. Her husband, Lucas, had qualities that were very different from those of her father, like the fact that he didn't drink, was more financially stable, and was more outgoing than her father ever was. But the repetition compulsion is a very powerful unconscious drive, and it can cause us to be blind to traits that are far more troublesome.

In Kelly's case, although her future husband appeared to be much more outgoing and accepting than her father ever was, when she got to know him better, she realized he was actually very critical of others, just as her father had been. But instead of seeing this as a red flag, Kelly saw it as a challenge. "I tried to discourage his critical behavior by mentioning something positive about the person he was critical of. Or I would say things like, 'I'll bet there is a good reason why that person acts that way.'"

Even though her future husband didn't change, she married him anyway. Because he wasn't directing his criticism at her, she convinced herself that it wasn't a real problem. Unfortunately, after they got married, her husband became increasingly critical of her, just as her father had been to her mother and to their children, including Kelly.

At this point in telling her story, Kelly broke down and cried. "I couldn't believe I'd married a man who was as critical as my father. I felt so stupid. How could I have made such a mistake?"

Even after Kelly became the target of her husband's constant criticism, she continued trying to change him with her positive attitude and outlook on life. But her husband just became more and more impatient with her and started calling her "Miss Pollyanna." Despite his refusal to change and the negative impact his criticalness had on Kelly's life, she ended up staying with him for ten long years. "I just took it, just like my mother had done," Kelly told me during one of our sessions. "I can't believe I did that."

If you suspect that perhaps you repeated a pattern from your parents' marriage or that you chose a partner because of the repetition compulsion, the following exercise will help you determine whether either or both are true for you.

DISCOVERING YOUR PATTERN

1. Draw a vertical line down the center of a piece of paper, making two columns.
2. In the left-side column, make a list of your ex-partner's emotional characteristics, both positive and negative (e.g., demanding, critical, good sense of humor).
3. Now, in the right-side column, write down the emotional characteristics (good and bad) of the person who was most abusive or neglectful toward you as you were growing up. It can be one of your parents or another family member or caretaker.
4. Read over your two lists and compare your answers. Circle the things the two people have in common.

This exercise can help you better recognize your pattern—the reasons why you were attracted to your ex-partner.

Other Reasons Why Your Past May Have Created Your Future

While repeating a pattern by replicating your parents' relationship or choosing a partner who is like one or both of your

parents is the most obvious reason for choosing an abusive partner, there are other life situations that can also influence our
choice of partner. For example, ask yourself, "What occurred in
my childhood, adolescence, or early adulthood that could have
had an impact on who I became attracted to or, conversely, who
was attracted to me?"

For example, if your mother or father emotionally or physically
abandoned you as a child, doesn't it make sense that you might
have been attracted to someone who wanted to be with you all
the time? Even if this person was overly possessive or jealous, isn't
it understandable that it might have felt good to have someone
care where you are all the time? Someone who couldn't bear to
be without you? Wouldn't this have comforted you since you are
always afraid of being abandoned again?

Or what if the opposite is true, what if you had a parent who
was emotionally smothering, engulfing, or controlling? Wouldn't
it make sense that you might be attracted to a partner who gave
you your freedom, who wasn't always around, who even needed
a lot of space himself? At first, this would have been a huge relief.
But as time went by, far from being smothering, your partner became aloof and distant and you seldom knew where he was. If you
asked him where he had been, he became defensive and accused
you of trying to "own him." What initially seemed like a healthy
relationship soon became a very unhealthy and unhappy one, with
you always feeling rejected and feeling guilty for behaving like
your smothering parent.

What if you were abused by someone other than a parent or
abused in other ways, such as sexual abuse? These traumas can
also influence who you chose as a partner.

Melinda was sexually abused by a neighbor from the time she
was eight years old until she was eleven. This abuse had a profound effect on how she felt about herself, primarily due to the
intense amount of shame she experienced. "For years I hated myself," she told me. "I thought the abuse was my fault because he

told me I had seduced him and because I kept going back. After all, if I didn't like it, why did I do that?"

> Because I felt so bad about myself I didn't think any man would want me. I wasn't popular in high school; in fact, boys pretty much ignored me. So when a guy at my first job started paying attention to me, I was pleasantly surprised. I was used to being passive, so it didn't bother me that he liked to be the one in charge of everything—like where we went and even what kind of sex we had. When he asked me to marry him, I was thrilled that anyone would even want me given how bad I felt about myself. That began almost fifteen years of utter hell, with my husband treating me like a slave and increasingly becoming more and more demanding sexually.
>
> I realize now that if I had not been sexually abused, I would have never married my husband. I would have realized that it isn't right for one partner to have total control over every aspect of the marriage. And I certainly wouldn't have given in to his outrageous and abusive sexual demands.

Some of you may be saying, "But I wasn't abused. My family life was pretty good. Why did *I* choose an abusive partner?" Sometimes, when people go through some kind of devastating loss (e.g., the death of a parent, a break-up or divorce), they become especially vulnerable, and in this state they can easily fall prey to an emotionally abusive person.

This is what my client Elena shared with me:

> I realize now that I would have never been attracted to my husband if I hadn't just lost my father. I was devastated, and this made me vulnerable to my husband's

charm. He swooped in and rescued me, holding me while I cried, listened to me as I talked endlessly about how much I missed my father. He was so kind and loving that I fell in love with him almost immediately. I didn't recognize that I was just trying to replace my father with another man.

Forgiving Yourself for the Harm You Caused Others

Forgiving yourself for the ways you have hurt or harmed others will probably be the hardest thing that you will ever have to do in order to heal your shame. In fact, it may be the hardest thing you ever have to do in your life. This is especially true if you have repeated the cycle of abuse by harming another person in the same ways you were harmed.

For example, it may seem impossible to forgive yourself for abusing your children. After all, you may know firsthand how much child abuse damages a child. And you probably know firsthand how much the shame that accompanies abuse can devastate a person's life. Here are some examples of what clients have shared with me regarding the shame they felt due to being abusive toward their children:

- "I remember how much it devastated me when my father criticized and shamed me. I can't believe I did that to my own child."
- "I promised myself I would not treat my children the way I was treated. And yet, to my horror, the very same words my mother said to me came out of my mouth. Those horrible, shaming, devastating words, 'I hate you. I wish you had never been born.' How can I forgive myself for saying those horrible words to the people I love most in the world?"

Understanding Why You Became a Neglectful or Abusive Parent

Victims of emotional abuse who have children often have a great deal of shame, not only for staying with the abuser but also for being a neglectful or abusive parent. If this is your situation, the following information will hopefully add to your understanding of why you behaved as you did toward your children.

First of all, remember that women and men who are being emotionally abused are being *traumatized*. These people use all of their focus and energy trying cope with this trauma, which can leave them unable to care for their children. They often walk around in a dissociated state or self-medicate with alcohol or drugs. This in turn can cause them to not notice when a child is upset or even when a child is in danger. This is what my client Hannah shared with me:

> When I was being abused, I didn't have the energy to
> be there for my children. It took all my energy to just
> get through the day. I didn't even notice when my old-
> est started taking drugs. I feel horrible about it,
> especially because my mother was never there for me.

Those who are being emotionally abused often carry a great deal of anger. Because you were likely afraid of your abusive partner, you probably held in that anger. But anger is the kind of emotion that needs to be expressed, and you may have ended up taking out your anger on your children. This is not to be construed as an excuse, merely an explanation. It is understandable that you would have inadvertently released your anger at your children.

In addition, research shows that the long-term effects of trauma tend to be the most obvious and prominent when people are stressed, in new situations, or in situations that remind them of the circumstances of their original trauma. Unfortunately, becoming a parent creates all three of these circumstances for someone who is being emotionally abused. First-time parenthood, in particular, is stressful and almost always triggers memories of our own childhood traumas. This can set the stage for child abuse.

The sad truth is that those who were abused or neglected in childhood are more likely to become abusive or neglectful of their own children than someone who didn't have these experiences. Traits that may have predisposed you to treat your children in abusive or neglectful ways include an inability to have compassion toward your child, a tendency to take things too personally (this may have caused you to overreact to your children's behavior by yelling, calling them names, or hitting them), being overly invested in your children looking good (and you looking good as their parent) due to your shame and lack of self-confidence, and an insistence on your children minding you or respecting you to compensate for your shame or lack of confidence.

And there is still another reason that can cause a parent to become abusive: seeing your own weakness or vulnerability in your child. Those with a history of having been victimized often develop a tendency to hate or despise weakness. If you saw weakness in your child, you may have been reminded of your own vulnerability and victimization, and this may have ignited your own self-hatred, thus causing you to lash out at your child.

Now that you have more understanding as to why you have acted as you have, you are more likely to be willing to forgive yourself for your negative actions and behaviors. If you continue to remind yourself that *it is understandable that you would have repeated the cycle of abuse given how you suffered as a child or how you were abused as an adult*, you will be able to take responsibility for your actions without further shaming yourself. Understanding that the traumas you experienced created problems within you that were out of your control can go a long way toward enabling you to forgive yourself for the ways that you have hurt others.

As Kristin Neff wrote in *Self-Compassion*, "When we begin to recognize that we are a product of countless factors, we don't need to take our 'personal failings' so personally. When we acknowledge the intricate web of causes and conditions in which we are all imbedded, we can be less judgmental of ourselves and others. A deep understanding of interconnectedness allows us to have compassion for the fact that we're doing the best we can given the hand life has dealt us."

UNDERSTANDING YOUR ACTIONS

1. Write a list of the people you have harmed and describe the ways you have harmed them.
2. One by one, go through your list and write down the various causes and conditions that led you to each action. In addition to the fact that you were abused as an adult and/or as a child, think of other precipitating factors, such as a family history of violence and a family history of addiction.
3. Now ask yourself why you didn't stop yourself from harming this person. For example, were you so full of rage that you couldn't control yourself? Did you hate yourself so much that you didn't care how much you hurt someone else? Had you built up such a defensive wall that you couldn't have empathy or compassion for the person you harmed?
4. Now that you have a better understanding of the causes and conditions that led you to act as you did, see if you feel more forgiving of yourself. You are an imperfect, fallible human being, and like all humans sometimes do, you acted in ways that hurt someone else. Honor the limitations of your human

imperfection. Have compassion for yourself. Forgive yourself.

If you find you are still overwhelmed with guilt or shame about how your past behavior has affected someone, it will be important to realize and remember this truth: *the most effective method of self-forgiveness is for you to vow that you will not continue the same behavior and not hurt someone in the same way again.*

Shame About Abusing Drugs or Alcohol

Many former victims of emotional abuse have tremendous shame due to the fact that they used drugs or alcohol to help them cope with the abuse. For example, my client Lena used alcohol to soothe the constant anxiety she experienced due to her husband's unrelenting criticism and unreasonable expectations.

> As soon as my husband left for work in the morning, I started drinking. At first I put just a little brandy in my coffee, telling myself I needed something to help me through the day. It relaxed me and allowed me to get the horrible names my husband called me out of my mind, at least temporarily.
>
> Then, as the time for my husband to come home drew closer, I started drinking vodka and orange juice to give me the courage to face him. I worried about whether the house was clean enough or if he'd like what I cooked him for dinner. I never knew what he'd find to criticize, but there was always something. If I was a little high, I was able to take it all without feeling destroyed. I could even pretend to love him. I could smile and be affectionate without a problem, and this

made him lay off me a little. Sometimes we got drunk together and even managed to have a good time.

But as time went by, I started drinking more and more, and he started noticing and making a big deal out of it. Now he could complain about having a lush for a wife. I knew I should stop drinking. I could see how it was affecting the way I treated our kids, and I hated myself for it. I especially hated myself for driving my kids around when I was drunk. I could have killed them.

When I first started working with Lena, she had managed to get away from her abusive husband, but she had lost custody of their three children. Her husband had used the fact that she had been given a DUI to try to blackmail her into staying with him. When that didn't work, he used the DUI against her in their child custody case.

Lena was extremely self-critical about the fact that she had become an alcoholic. "I'm so stupid. How could I have done this to myself—and my children?"

I explained to her that she was far from being stupid. In fact, she had found a very clever (albeit self-destructive) way to self-medicate. Once I explained to Lena that she actually had a good reason to drink and that she was doing the best she could to cope with the emotional abuse, she became less critical of herself. I then explained to her that while getting drunk helped her to cope with the abuse, this coping mechanism was maladaptive in that it did not help her heal from the abuse. In fact, her drinking resulted in more trauma (i.e., the loss of her children).

I am happy to report that thanks to counseling and Alcoholics Anonymous, Lena has been sober for two years now. She has also gained the strength and self-esteem to fight for custody of her children and has won that battle.

If you have an alcohol or drug dependency, it is important to realize that it is very likely that you are using the substance to cope with either the emotional abuse or a history of child abuse or both. Most important, understand that your addiction—whether it be to alcohol, drugs, sex, food, shopping, or gambling —has been a way to self-medicate and to cope with anxiety and fear. This can help you to stop beating yourself up for the harm your addiction caused to those close to you.

IT IS UNDERSTANDABLE

- Make a list of the ways you have coped with being emotionally abused. For example, maybe you isolated yourself from others because you felt such shame for putting up with the abuse, or maybe you began to drink more heavily as a way of coping with the abuse.
- For each of the coping mechanisms you used, tell yourself, "It is understandable." For example: "It is understandable that I pushed my friends away. I felt so much shame. I couldn't imagine they could accept me if they knew what was happening. " Or, "It is understandable that I started drinking more as a way of coping with my pain."

Forgiving Yourself for the Harm You Caused Yourself

Although you may have a hard time believing it, forgiving yourself for the harm you caused yourself is just as important as forgiving yourself for the harm you brought to others. Sometimes this harm is obvious—the harm you have done to your body due to excessive drinking, drugs, cigarettes, overeating or eating unhealthy foods; purging and bingeing; self-mutilation; having un-protected sex or promiscuous sex.

Forgive yourself for indulging in these behaviors. You didn't love and respect your body because of the massive amounts of shame you carried. You hated your body because it was a source of pain and shame. You starved your body because you had been starved of love, nurturing, and proper care when you were a child or by your abusive partner. You attacked your body because others had attacked it and you felt that this was what it deserved. You were reckless with your body because no one had cherished it when you were growing up.

Forgive yourself for the things you did that damaged your spirit, your image of yourself, and your integrity. Forgive yourself for going along with your partner's abusive or even unlawful be-havior; forgive yourself for allowing your partner to force you into engaging in sex acts that felt repulsive or disgusting to you; forgive yourself for turning your back on family and friends who loved you and who were worried about you.

Often, the harm you have caused yourself is subtler than the obvious harm you did to your body, your self-esteem, or your self-image. For example, you need to forgive yourself for not believing in yourself, for being too hard on yourself, for blaming yourself for the abuse, and for setting unreasonable expectations for your-self. Remember that you were doing the best you could at the time, that you didn't know any other way to be, and that you were just doing what you had been taught to do.

You pushed people away because you were afraid to trust, be-cause you didn't believe you deserved to be loved. You didn't believe in yourself because no one had believed in you as you were growing up and because your abuser told you lies about yourself that you believed instead. You were too hard on yourself, and you set unreasonable expectations of yourself because others were too hard on you, including your parents and your abuser.

SELF-FORGIVENESS LETTER

1. Write a letter asking yourself for forgiveness. Include all the ways you have harmed yourself, including ways that you have neglected your body and ways that you have treated yourself like your parents or abusers treated you. Also include ways you have harmed yourself by being too hard on yourself.

2. Don't expect yourself to write this letter in one sitting. It may take several days or even weeks to complete it. Take your time and carefully consider the many ways you have harmed yourself.

3. As you write, bring up all the self-compassion you can muster. If you begin to feel self-critical, stop writing. Either do one of the other self-compassion exercises in the book or reread a portion of the book that will remind you of why you acted the way you did. Then and only then, go back to your letter with self-compassion in your heart and mind.

HEART MEDITATION: FORGIVING YOURSELF FOR THE WAYS YOU HAVE HARMED YOURSELF

1. Sit comfortably, allowing your eyes to close and your breath to be natural and easy.

2. Let your body and mind relax.

3. Breathe gently into the area of your heart, and let yourself feel all the barriers you have erected and

the emotions that you have carried because you haven't forgiven yourself.

4. Let your heart feel the pain of keeping your heart closed.

5. (Breathing) Breathe softly and begin extending forgiveness toward yourself, reciting the following words: "There are many ways that I have hurt or harmed myself. I have betrayed or abandoned myself many times through thought, word, or deed, knowingly or unknowingly."

6. Feel your own precious body and life. Let yourself see the ways you have hurt or harmed yourself.

7. Feel the sorrow you have carried from this. Sense that you can release these burdens.

8. Extend forgiveness to each of these burdens, one by one.

9. Repeat to yourself: "For the ways I have hurt myself through action or inaction, out of shame, fear, pain, or anger, I now extend a full and heartfelt forgiveness. I forgive myself, I forgive myself."

Forgiving yourself will do more for you in terms of healing your shame than almost anything you can do. Forgive yourself for the abuse itself. You were an innocent victim who did not deserve to be abused. Forgive yourself for the ways you reenacted the abuse. You were full of shame, and as you have learned, shame causes us to do horrendous things to ourselves and others.

If you were traumatized as a child, forgive yourself for the way it negatively affected your ability to choose a healthy partner. Forgive yourself for being so insecure, for having such low self-esteem, for feeling so much shame, for being so afraid of rejection or abandonment that you took what you could get. Forgive yourself for wanting to undo the past by trying to recreate it.

Forgive yourself for staying because you were so afraid of being alone. Forgive yourself for repeating your mother's or your father's behavior by staying with an abusive partner. Forgive yourself for following your family's or your church's belief that divorce is never acceptable. Forgive yourself for believing, like one or both of your parents did, that people can change if you are just patient enough. Forgive yourself for all this and more.

CHAPTER 15

Continue to Focus on Healing Your Shame

Go back and take care of yourself. Your body needs you, your feelings need you, your perceptions need you. Your suffering needs you to acknowledge it. Go home and be there for all these things.

—THICH NHAT HANH, *Reconciliation: Healing the Inner Child*

SHAME CARVES DEEP SCARS in people who have endured emotional abuse. These scars include damage to your core perception of yourself and your identity, continuing to be overwhelmed with feelings of disgust and humiliation, and continuing to chastise yourself for putting up with the abuse. You, like many former victims, may be haunted by the realization that you put up with abuse for too long, the shame of having kept the secret from friends and family, and the continuing tendency to question whether the failure of the relationship was somehow your fault. If this isn't enough, shame can poison your belief in yourself, including your belief that you can make it on your own, your belief that anyone will ever love you again, and the belief that you are capable of choosing a healthy, safe partner in the future.

All this shame needs to be healed. It needs to be addressed head-on and banished from your body, mind, and spirit. In this chapter, I will offer more ways for you to accomplish this healing. We will also focus on more ways for you to continue learning and practicing self-compassion, including more specific compassionate attitudes and skills that can reverse your tendency to view yourself in blaming, condemning, and self-critical ways. This will require you to continue to work on all aspects of self-compassion: *self-understanding, self-forgiveness, self-acceptance, self-kindness, and self-encouragement.*

Healing Your Body of Shame

Why do you need to heal your body of shame? One important reason is that our body communicates with us and to others how we feel about ourselves. Our posture is one clear indication of how we feel about ourselves. Trauma experts such as Peter Levine have been working with clients on helping them change their posture from the typical shame posture of slumping their shoulders, curling their chest in, and keeping their head down to a more empowering one of head up, chest out, and shoulders back, and they have found it effective in helping clients eliminate shame and feel more empowered.

The following body exercise will help you begin to change your posture, which in turn can help you change your emotions and your mind.

Taking the Shame Out of your Posture

 1. Sit in a chair the way you normally do. If you can sit in front of a mirror, that is ideal, but it isn't

necessary. Notice your posture. Are you slumped over, or are you sitting straight? Are your shoulders pulled back, or are they slumped forward, almost as if they are protecting your chest area?

2. Notice how your posture makes you feel. Do you feel low-energy? Do you feel passive?

3. Now I'd like you to pull your shoulders back and sit up straighter. Imagine that there is an imaginary string attached to your head and that someone is pulling on the string and making your head lift. Take deep breaths and expand your chest, almost like you are Tarzan pounding his chest. With each deep breath, notice how your chest feels like it is opening up.

4. Notice how you feel now. Do you sense any difference in how you feel emotionally when you sit up straighter, when you expand your chest? If you are sitting near a mirror, notice how your appearance has changed.

Here are some remarks some of my clients have made about the differences they felt:

· "I felt taller when I sat up straighter, and for some reason this made me feel stronger, less afraid."
· "I noticed I was slumping before, but when I pulled my shoulders back I felt more confident. I even felt more assertive."
· "I felt powerful when I opened my chest area and took some deep breaths. With each breath, it felt like I was becoming more and more confident."

Shame Memories

Current research has shown that we can actually rewire our shame memories. Given the neural plasticity of the brain—the capacity of our brains to grow new neurons and new synaptic connections lifelong—you can proactively repair old shame memories with new experiences of self-empathy and self-compassion. We do this by evoking an old shame memory—activating those well-rehearsed neural networks. Then we cultivate *self-empathy* and *self-compassion* so that now *those* neural networks are firing. The two patterns of neural networks—those evoked by the shame memory and those evoked by self-empathy and self-compassion— are now firing together. New circuitry is created in that moment, sometimes quite dramatically. The sense of shame literally dissolves in the larger self-awareness and self-compassion, much like a teaspoon of salt in a lake. There is no more charge. Obviously, this will need to be practiced over and over in cases in which someone has been repeatedly shamed, but eventually it works. The following exercise is an example of how this works.

REWIRING YOUR SHAME MEMORIES

1. Place your hand on your heart and breathe deeply.
2. Evoke a memory of being loved.
3. Allow yourself to feel the feelings of being loved flow through your mind and body.
4. Now bring forth a small segment of an old memory of shame, a teaspoonful, not a large amount.
5. Hold that memory of shame in the larger awareness of your goodness, strength, and wisdom. Hold it in the larger context of the love and acceptance of others and of the growing amount of love and ac-

ceptance you feel toward yourself. You may even feel a sense of a shift in your body as your whole body begins to deeply encode this new way of being, feeling, and thinking.

I encourage you to repeat this practice of repairing as many times as is necessary to rewire the old neural wiring of shame.

Continue to Practice Self-Compassion

Continuing to practice self-compassion is the most powerful way for you to heal your shame. In addition to self-compassion being the antidote to shame, it can also act as an antidote to self-criticism—a major tendency of those who experience intense shame. Research has found that self-compassion is a powerful trigger for the release of oxytocin, the hormone that increases feelings of trust, calmness, safety, generosity, and connectedness. Self-criticism, on the other hand, has a very different effect on our body. The amygdala, the oldest part of the brain, is designed to quickly detect threats in the environment. When we experience a threatening situation, the fight-or-flight response is triggered and the amygdala sends signals that increase blood pressure, adrenaline, and the hormone cortisol, mobilizing the strength and energy we need to confront or avoid the threat. Although our bodies created this system to deal with physical attacks, it is activated just as readily by emotional attacks—from within and without. Over time, increased cortisol levels lead to depression because they deplete the various neurotransmitters that allow us to experience pleasure.

One of the many benefits of practicing self-compassion is that it releases oxytocin into our body. The following exercise will show you ways to use this oxytocin.

USING OXYTOCIN

Bring to mind someone you love, someone you unconditionally love. This could be a dear friend, a beloved child or
pet, or someone who has offered you love and support, such
as a therapist.

1. Feel the love you feel for this person or pet in your
   body. Notice how it feels. Sense the flow of love
   from you to your loved one.
2. After you've connected to this feeling of love, allow
   the flow of love that you have been sending in your
   loved one's direction to begin to come back to you.
   Continue to feel the empathy and love you feel for
   your loved one, but let it flow back to yourself.
3. If you can, let yourself receive this love and empathy; receive the care, the feeling of being loved and
   cared for by yourself.

The Importance of Validation

There is still another benefit that comes from self-compassion: validation. Put simply, to validate is to confirm. Validation is
recognizing and accepting that another person's internal experience matters. When someone validates another's experience, the
message that is sent is, "Your feelings make sense. Not only do I
hear you, I also understand why you feel as you do. You are not
bad or wrong or crazy for feeling the way you do."

On the other hand, to invalidate means to attack or question
the foundation or reality of a person's feelings. This can be done
through denying, ridiculing, ignoring, or judging another per-

son's feelings. Regardless of the method, the effect is clear: the person feels "wrong." Because of this, it is vitally important that your perceptions and your feelings are validated today. Having self-compassion, connecting to one's own suffering, is a way of validating yourself, your feelings, your perceptions, and your experiences.

It is often lack of validation that contributes to the development of feelings of guilt and shame as a reaction to negative experiences. For example, if you are like most victims of emotional abuse, you likely have not told anyone about the abuse. Because of this, your experience of the abuse itself has likely never been validated. In order to heal from the abuse and the shame surrounding it, it is important that you receive validation now—from yourself and others.

Self-compassion will help you give yourself the nurturance, understanding, and validation you so desperately need in order to heal your shame and begin to feel worthy of care and acceptance.

The Compassionate Letter

I asked my client Maureen to write a "compassionate letter" to herself in which she offered herself compassion for all she'd suffered as a result of the emotional abuse she experienced while married to her husband of twenty years. This is what she wrote:

> I am so sorry you have suffered so much in your marriage. It must have been unbearable to put up with that abuse for so many years. You must have felt so trapped and so alone. I know you were afraid to tell anyone what was happening to you because you were afraid they wouldn't believe you or they would reject you. And since you loved your husband and he was a good father and a good provider, I know you felt guilty just

thinking about leaving him. Your husband did so many
terrible things to you and said such horrible things to
you, and I wish this wouldn't have happened to you.
And I wish there had been someone there to comfort
you after each and every one of these traumas. You suffered from depression and self-blame afterwards, and
you became more and more numb. You didn't deserve
to be treated like this.

As you will notice, not only did Maureen offer herself comfort
and understanding for her suffering in this letter, she also *validated*
her feelings.

A study conducted by two researchers, Leah B. Shapira and
Myriam Mongrain, found that adults who wrote a compassionate
letter to themselves once a day for a week acknowledging the distressing events they had experienced showed significant
reductions in depression over three months and significant increases in happiness over six months, compared with members of
a control group who were asked to write about early memories.

In addition to validating yourself, you also need to be validated
by others. I encourage you to tell someone you trust about the
fact that you have been emotionally abused. I know it is scary. You
may have tried this before and found that the person didn't believe you or tried to talk you out of trusting your own experience.
But you are stronger now, and you don't need someone else believing you in order to know what reality is. You do, however, need
to step out of your isolation and discover whether there are those
around you who will believe and support you. One of the best
places to receive this support is in a group for people who are
being emotionally abused. Find out if such a group exists in your
community. Check with your local battered women's organization.
Many offer support groups, not only for women who are being
physically abused but also for those who are being or have been
emotionally abused as well. Meetup is also a popular option.

There are groups in the United States, Scotland, Canada, Australia, and New Zealand. Go to abuse.meetup.com for more information. Although they are not an optimal choice, there are also online groups and forums on emotional abuse.

Moving from Self-Criticism to Self-Acceptance

In addition to having a powerful inner critic, former victims of emotional abuse often have unreasonable expectations of themselves. The emotional abuse you suffered probably included your partner having unreasonable expectations of you. Because of this, it is highly likely that you may have taken on this same behavior toward yourself. You likely expect yourself to always do things correctly and not make mistakes. And when you do make the inevitable mistake or behave inappropriately, you are likely very unforgiving of yourself. You may chastise yourself just as harshly as your abuser did, or you may even punish yourself by starving yourself, depriving yourself of anything good, or inflicting self-harm.

For this reason, it is important to begin to have more reasonable expectations of yourself—expectations that are neither too harsh nor too lenient. If you don't do this, you will inevitably set yourself up to feel disappointed in yourself (and activate your critical inner voice). A reasonable expectation is one that is reachable, given your history, your present situation, and who you are today. For example, it is *reasonable* that given your history of being abused, you likely suffer from low self-esteem, a strong inner critic, and unhealthy shame. It is *unreasonable* to expect that given your history you would be able to overcome these negative effects of abuse overnight. It is *reasonable*, however, to expect that by reading this book and doing the exercises, you may be able to overcome much of the damage you suffered.

IT IS MORE REASONABLE

1. Think of a current behavior that you would like to change (e.g., be a better parent).
2. Using the format below, fill in the blanks.

   Given the fact that _____, it is unreasonable that I _____.

   It is more reasonable that I _____.

Example: "Given the fact that my parents were so critical of me, it is unreasonable that I will never be critical of my own children. It is more reasonable that I can catch myself when I am being critical, acknowledge this to myself and my children, and continue to work on not being critical."

Stop Expecting Yourself to Be "All Good"

Another way that you may have set unreasonable expectations for yourself is by expecting yourself to always be respectful, generous, patient, kind, and forgiving—in other words, to be "all good." But the truth is, no one can be good all the time. We all have times when we feel petty or small-minded, we can all be selfish, and we all become angry at times. If we accept this fact, we can forgive ourselves of our shortcomings, vow to do better, and move on. If we expect ourselves to never be petty or selfish and to never get angry, we are setting ourselves up for feeling shame.

The truth is, we cannot put aside our less acceptable traits such as selfishness or a tendency to be mean or to get angry without these very traits rearing their ugly heads eventually. And those who try to be all good often have an investment in looking good and doing good deeds because they carry so much shame.

This can set one up to be codependent or to put up with unacceptable behavior in others. It is as if people hope that by doing good they will erase any bad things they have done in their lives. How about you? Do you have an investment in being all good in order to compensate for the amount of shame that you carry?

THE POWER OF INQUIRY

This exercise is based on the mindfulness practice called *inquiry*. Try it the next time you behave in a way that upsets you, such as yelling at one of your children or engaging in behaviors such as overeating.

1. Pause and ask yourself, "What inside me needs the most attention?" or "What wants to be accepted?" This will help you drop below your self-judgment and help you connect with your emotions.
2. Notice what is going on in your body. Are the muscles in your stomach contracted? Is the rest of your body tight? If so, ask yourself what emotions you might be feeling to cause your body to be so tight. You might be feeling fear—perhaps the fear of failing or of not being a good parent.
3. Notice how just paying attention to the emotion of fear can cause it to diminish, and with it, the self-judgment.
4. Now add compassion to your practice of mindful inquiry. Send a message to the emotion of fear (or pain, or anger, or shame): "I care about this suffering." Sit with your feelings like you would sit with a good friend who is struggling. Repeat the words "I care about this suffering" several times.

The attitude of self-acceptance exemplified in this exercise makes it safe for the frightened and vulnerable parts of your being to let themselves be known. The practice of self-compassion will help you to stop striving for perfection in yourself and, instead, learn how to love yourself into wholeness.

Tara Bach, in her wonderful book *Radical Acceptance: Embracing Your Life with the Heart of a Buddha*, suggests we take on the attitude that we are already perfect just the way we are—shortcomings and all. You don't need to continually strive to become a better version of yourself; you are already wonderful. Just as a good parent loves and accepts her child just as he is, strive to love and accept yourself just as you are.

RADICAL ACCEPTANCE

1. Make a list of your flaws: aspects of yourself you are ashamed of, aspects of yourself you have been working on changing.
2. Read each flaw out loud, and then say to yourself, "May I love and accept myself just as I am." Take a deep breath each time you say this phase, and really take it in.
3. Know that every aspect of yourself belongs and is acceptable.

Above all, realize that everyone longs to be accepted for who they are. Most of us have spent our life seeking validation and approval from others. But the truth is, if we cannot accept ourselves, we cannot expect others to accept us. And without self-acceptance, we will live in constant fear of being rejected.

The opposite of acceptance is rejection. If you do not accept yourself fully, you are implicitly rejecting some part of yourself. When you deny, repress, or hide any aspect of yourself, it is akin to rejecting yourself. If you walk around hiding certain aspects, disguising who you really are, you shrink and live a partial life. On the other hand, if you own all your qualities and life experiences, you flourish and expand into wholeness.

Self-Kindness

We began our discussion of self-kindness in chapter 8. *Self-kindness*, a major component of *self-compassion*, is one of the most powerful ways of healing your shame. In fact, self-kindness is the heart of self-compassion. Unfortunately, you may have no idea how to practice it. Self-kindness involves viewing yourself and treating yourself in a tender, loving, gentle manner. It is about adopting an attitude of kindness, patience, and self-acceptance toward yourself versus an attitude of self-criticism, perfectionism, and unreasonable expectations.

It also involves generating feelings of care and comfort toward oneself. Instead of being self-critical, self-kindness involves being tolerant of our flaws and inadequacies. This includes learning simple tools for giving ourselves the support we need whenever we suffer, fail, or feel inadequate.

Being kind to oneself can come naturally to those who believe they deserve it. Unfortunately, your shame has probably kept you from feeling kind toward yourself in much the same way that it may have made it difficult for you to accept kindness from others. Hopefully, with some of your shame dissipated, you will now be more open to believing you deserve self-kindness. However, I do understand that it will be more difficult for some. It is often difficult to learn to treat yourself with kindness if you haven't experienced much kindness from others. As mentioned earlier, it often helps to mimic the way one of the people who have been kind to you treated you. But even if you don't know how to treat yourself with loving kindness, if you now believe you deserve it, then the information and suggestions here will help you learn how to practice it.

In some ways, you have already begun to learn how to practice self-kindness, since stopping the constant self-judgment and self-criticism that you have been used to and coming to understand, accept, and forgive your weaknesses and mistakes instead of condemning them are all part of self-kindness

There is neurological evidence showing that self-kindness and self-criticism operate quite differently in terms of brain function. A recent study found that self-criticism was associated with activity in the lateral prefrontal cortex and the dorsal anterior cingulate cortex—areas of the brain associated with error processing and problem solving. Being kind and reassuring toward oneself, on the other hand, was associated with activation of the left temporal pole and the insula—areas of the brain associated with positive emotions and compassion. Instead of seeing ourselves as a problem to be fixed, therefore, self-kindness allows us to see ourselves as valuable human beings who are worthy of care.

Practicing self-kindness will motivate you to take better care of yourself, including making sure you are safe and not doing anything that will jeopardize your safety and integrity. It will also help you make wiser and healthier choices, including choosing to act in healthier ways.

If you don't love yourself and have a deep desire to honor yourself and your values, then you will continue to be passive when you don't want to be. But when you can put your need to be safe and to be treated with respect ahead of other less important needs, such as always trying to please your partner, then you will find that you'll respect yourself far more.

Supporting Yourself

It is often easier to tolerate difficult feelings and situations if we feel supported by others. The same is true when it comes to our relationship with ourselves. The kinder and more compassionate we are with ourselves, the more we can develop the courage to tolerate difficult things. The following exercise is yet another way to connect with your emotions related to the abuse and to provide support and nurturing toward yourself.

PICTURE YOURSELF

If you have pictures of yourself as a child, please go through them and find one or two that resonate with you, pictures that remind you of your childhood. If you can find a picture of yourself when you were going through a particularly difficult time (e.g., your parents got a divorce, you were sexually abused) that would be ideal.

1. Take a long look at the picture or pictures you have chosen.
2. Notice the expression on your face, your posture, and any other cues that might be present to show how you were feeling at the time. You may notice that you look sad, afraid, or angry. On the other hand, you may not be able to see any cues.
3. Notice how you feel as you look at the pictures and as you think about what you were going through at the time.
4. Write yourself a letter telling your child self how you feel now as you think about how you suffered

as a child. Write it as if your adult self is addressing
your child self.

5. Once you have completed your letter, read it out
loud to yourself (or more accurately, to your child
self). Allow yourself to take in these words of kindness, support, and compassion.

Learning Ways to Self-Soothe

Self-soothing is actually something many children learn to
provide for themselves as part of a natural developmental
stage. It goes like this: A child begins to cry out for her mother.
A responsive mother reacts quickly to her child's cries. She
picks up her baby and soothes her with a gentle voice and
touch. She ascertains what it is that her baby needs, whether it
is food, a diaper change, or simply to be held and comforted.
This is considered an *empathetic response*, which makes the
baby feel safe and reassured. From experiences like this, an
infant learns in a deeply unconscious way that she can get
what she needs, when she needs it, and that all will be okay.
This unconscious experience of knowing that she will be
responded to adequately and that everything will be taken
care of translates into the ability to *self-soothe*.

You may have noticed that when life presents challenges, you
often experience an intensity of distress that feels excessive and
out of control. Or you may experience a depth of hopelessness
and futility that seems overwhelmingly powerful. If this is true for
you, it may be because your needs were not responded to in a
soothing, nurturing way when you were an infant or toddler. It
may also mean that as an infant or toddler you experienced a great

deal of interpersonal chaos (such as often hearing your parents fighting), parental neglect, or rage. All these experiences would have created an intense anxiety inside of you as a child. This does not mean that you will never feel comfortable and confident about getting your needs met and never be able to self-soothe, however. In fact, the following information and exercises can help you begin to repair these deficits.

Soothing Your Pain Through Gentle Touch and Hugging

Imagine how it would have felt if there had been someone available to hold you or gently rock you after each experience of being emotionally abused by your partner. Being lovingly cared for in this way would not have made the abuse go away, but it would have soothed your pain in the moment. Although you probably did not receive this kind of loving touch at the time, it is not too late to provide it for yourself as you go through this grieving and healing process.

1. As you remember the pain of an abuse experience or a memory of the abuse is triggered by something in your environment, try each of the following: (1) gently stroke your arm, face, or hair, (2) gently rock your body, or (3) give yourself a warm hug.
2. Notice how your body feels after receiving each of these self-soothing techniques. Does it feel calmer, more relaxed?
3. Notice which of these self-soothing techniques feels the best to you. For example, do you have more positive associations with one rather than the other?

4. Don't allow your self-critical mind to try to talk you out of this. It is not silly or self-centered to soothe yourself; it is a loving thing to do for yourself.

There is actual research that shows that the power of self-kindness is not just some feel-good idea that doesn't really change things. For example, one important way that self-soothing works is by triggering the release of oxytocin, which researchers have dubbed the "hormone of love and bonding." I mentioned the research on oxytocin earlier in this chapter and discussed how the hormone has been shown to increase feelings of trust, calm, safety, generosity, and connectedness and to also facilitate the ability to feel warmth and compassion for ourselves. This is especially true when you self-soothe by touching your body in a gentle way because physical touch releases oxytocin, which has been shown to reduce fear and anxiety and to counteract the increased blood pressure and cortisol associated with stress.

There are many ways to physically soothe yourself. Many of my clients find that softly stroking their cheeks or gently stroking their arms is especially comforting. Find a way that works for you to soothe yourself through touch.

Provide for Yourself What You Need

Another aspect of self-kindness is providing for yourself what you need and want in life—not just when you are in distress, but overall. In order to do this, you must be self-aware. Self-awareness involves learning about yourself—paying attention to yourself, including your feelings and your reactions. There are many examples of how, by not being self-aware, we put ourselves in situations or force ourselves to do things that we don't really want to do. Think about how often you put your own needs aside in order to do what you think is expected of you or in order to please someone else.

Become Your Own Nurturing and Responsive Parent

Since you are likely the victim of some kind of childhood abuse or neglect, it is highly likely that you did not have a nurturing and responsive parent. One or both of your parents may have been re-enacting their own childhood abuse by neglecting or abusing you, or your parents may not have known how to meet your emotional needs. Or perhaps your parents may have been too preoccupied with making a living to attend to your emotional needs. For any and all of these reasons, it will be important for you to become your own nurturing and responsive parent today.

Laurel Mellin, in her outstanding book and program *The Pathway: Follow the Road to Health and Happiness*, explains that in order to become your own responsive parent, you need to create a balance between the two extremes of depriving yourself and indulging yourself. This middle point is called *responsiveness*. As we discussed earlier in this chapter, a responsive parent is keenly aware of her child's needs. If her baby cries and it isn't readily obvious why he is doing so, she makes every effort to discover what his needs are. She doesn't change her baby's diapers when the baby is crying because it is hungry. Neither does she try to feed her baby when what the child really needs is to be held. When a responsive parent discovers and fulfills her child's real needs, she doesn't need to indulge the child. She doesn't need to make up for any neglectful treatment on her part. She knows she has been responsive to her child's real needs and doesn't suffer from guilt or shame feelings.

Just as a responsive parent is aware of her child's needs, you need to become aware of and sensitive to your own needs. Once you have identified your real needs, you will have more of an ability to meet them. Unfortunately, discovering our real needs is not usually that easy, especially if you had depriving or overly permissive parents.

The Connection Between Needs and Feelings

One way of discovering what your needs are at any given time is to check in with your feelings. Your feelings will tell you what you need if you pay close attention. The following exercise will help you make this important connection.

FEELINGS AND NEEDS

1. Check in with yourself several times a day by "going inside" and asking yourself what you are feeling. It is sometimes easier to stick with the four basic feelings of anger, sadness, fear, and guilt or shame. Ask yourself, "Am I feeling angry?" If the answer is no, you would go on to "Am I feeling sad?' and so on. You may find that your answer to "What am I feeling?" may also be something like "lonely" or "hungry."

2. When you find a feeling, look for the corresponding need. Ask yourself, "What do I need?" Often, the answer will be "Feel my feeling and let it fade." Keep it simple; don't confuse the issue with too many details or complexities. For example, when you feel angry, you may need to speak up for yourself. When you feel sad, you may need to cry. If you are hungry, you need food. When you feel guilty, you need to apologize.

3. It may take trying on several needs before you find the one that is true for you. You may also have

many needs attached to one feeling. For example, you may feel lonely and your needs may be to call a friend, get a hug from your partner, and connect with yourself.

4. Be on the alert for answers that are not truly responsive to you; for example, if you feel sad and your "need" is to get some candy, or if you feel angry so you "need" to hit somebody. Instead, tap into your inherent wisdom and relax into a more logical, self-nurturing answer. Ask yourself, "Okay, what do I really need?" Some more logical, constructive needs may be "Express myself (write, sing)," "Get physical (walk, stomp)," "Develop a plan," or "Learn from it (for the next time)."

As you continue to practice self-kindness, you may experience a phenomenon in which you are inundated with intense feelings of grief or other negative emotions or traumatic or painful memories. Your old core beliefs about yourself from childhood ("I'm unlovable," "I'm worthless") may also emerge as you make the practice of self-kindness more a part of your life.

My wise and compassionate therapist explained this phenomenon to me in this way: When we first start working on our issues, we are like a vessel filled with feelings of shame, pain, anger, fear, and guilt. As we begin to heal, especially as we start to provide ourselves with self-compassion and self-kindness, it is as if we are pouring this kindness and compassion into that vessel. Since the vessel is already full of shame and other negative emotions, we must make room for the new positive feelings of self-kindness and love. What happens is that our shame and other negative emotions start pouring out in order to make room for the feelings of self-kindness and love. For example, the more kind and compassionate you are to yourself, the more feelings of grief for all the times you felt alone and misunderstood may come pouring out.

The way to deal with this predictable situation is to address it directly and not try to push away the bad feelings. You can say, "I've been feeling really good about myself, so it makes sense (or it is *understandable*) that old feelings of self-doubt and self-hatred might come up."

If feelings such as grief become intense, don't panic; just allow the feelings to come forth. Allow yourself to grieve for all the past times when you were in pain and there was no one there to comfort you. In other words, be gentle with yourself and comfort yourself in your pain and suffering.

It will take time and practice to make self-kindness a natural part of your life. But you can learn to listen to your needs and honor them. You can learn to stop ignoring your body's signals (e.g., for rest, for healthy food) and instead respond to them. And by developing the ability to self-soothe, you also learn to love yourself even when you make mistakes.

The good news is that there is a self-rewarding aspect to self-kindness. Every day provides you a new opportunity to meet your suffering with kindness, and every time you do this you are deepening your belief that you deserve such kindness. The more you respond to yourself in a kind way when you make a mistake or when things go wrong, the more you erase the damage you experienced from years of self-criticism (or criticism from others). The more you soothe and nurture yourself when you feel sad, afraid, angry, or guilty, the less you will tend to become overwhelmed by your less-than-positive emotions.

Above all, remember this: You deserve to be kind to yourself. You deserve to soothe yourself when you are stressed. You deserve to know and meet your basic needs for rest, good nutrition, and connection with others—needs that every human being has.

CONCLUSION

Moving Forward

The very least you can do in life is figure out what you hope for. And the most you can do is live inside that hope. Not admire it from a distance but live right in it, under its roof.

—BARBARA KINGSOLVER, *Animal Dreams*

YOU AND I HAVE BEEN on a long journey together—an expedition, really. The purpose of this expedition was to discover whether you were being emotionally abused and just how this abuse has affected you. But another, equally important purpose was to help you rediscover yourself—to help you remember who you were before you met your partner, who you were before you were so deeply shamed.

No matter where you are at this point—whether you have ended your relationship or are still considering it, whether you are actively preparing yourself to leave or have decided to stay and try to make it work—my deepest hope is that this book has helped you to heal your shame, most especially the shame you've been experiencing because of the way your partner has treated you.

I hope you have come to acknowledge the suffering you've experienced due to your partner's abuse and have learned how to practice self-compassion. Even if you aren't prepared to end your relationship, I hope you are determined to find a way to take better care of yourself and to honor your feelings.

There has been a lot of information in this book—a lot of processes and exercises, a lot of requests for you to be open to changing your mind, your feelings, and your beliefs. Even though it has no doubt been difficult, hopefully, you've experienced a lot of changes, the most important being developing a stronger belief that you deserve to be treated with respect, consideration, and kindness.

You've learned that self-compassion is the antidote to shame. You've learned that anger pushes away shame. And you've learned that self-forgiveness is the healing balm you need to heal your wounds and your shame. But there is one more thing you need to learn: pride is the opposite of self-blame and shame. At this point, it is important that you acknowledge how much you have grown, how much courage it took to end your emotionally abusive relationship, and any other positive changes you have created. Let yourself remember where you started from and then give yourself credit for how far you've come. Be proud of yourself. You deserve it.

It has taken a lot of work on your part to make these changes and a lot of courage to persist in the process. I commend you for your courage and for your strength. You are far more courageous and strong than you realize—a lot more.

You can go on from here to become an even stronger and more courageous person—a person who will not let anyone shame you, manipulate you, or control you again. A person who can begin your life again, wounded but not destroyed.

It has been an honor and a privilege to walk beside you on your journey. I will keep you in my heart, and I hope you will keep me in yours.

I will leave you with this quote:

> *Sometimes the strength within you is not a big fiery flame for all to see. It is just a tiny spark that whispers ever so softly, "You got this. Keep going."*
>
> —ANONYMOUS

Recommended Reading

Recovery from Trauma

Herman, Judith Lewis. *Trauma and Recovery: The Aftermath of Violence—From Domestic Abuse to Political Terror.*

Levine, Peter. *Healing Trauma: A Pioneering Program for Restoring the Wisdom of Your Body.*

Recovery from Childhood Abuse and Neglect

Engel, Beverly. *Healing Your Emotional Self: A Powerful Program to Help You Raise Your Self-Esteem, Quiet Your Inner Critic, and Overcome Shame.*

———. *It Wasn't Your Fault: Freeing Yourself from the Shame of Childhood Abuse with the Power of Self-Compassion.*

Forward, Susan. *Mothers Who Can't Love: A Healing Guide for Daughters.*

McBride, Karyl. *Will I Ever Be Enough? Healing the Daughters of Narcissistic Mothers.*

Recovery from Sexual Abuse and Assault

Atkinson, Matt. *Resurrection After Rape: A Guide to Transforming from Victim to Survivor.*

Bass, Ellen, and Davis, Laura. *The Courage to Heal: A Guide for Women Survivors of Child Sexual Abuse.*

Lew, Mike. *Victims No Longer: The Classic Guide for Men Recovering from Sexual Child Abuse.*

Recovery from Emotional Abuse (in Adulthood)

Engel, Beverly. *The Emotionally Abused Woman: Overcoming Destructive Patterns and Reclaiming Yourself.*
_____. *The Emotionally Abusive Relationship: How to Stop Being Abused and How to Stop Abusing.*
Evans, Patricia. *The Verbally Abusive Relationship.*
Forward, Susan. *Emotional Blackmail: When the People in Your Life Use Fear, Obligation, and Guilt to Manipulate You.*

Recovery from Codependency

Lancer, Darlene. *Conquering Shame and Codependency: 8 Steps to Freeing the True You.*

Anger

Engel, Beverly. *Honor Your Anger: How Transforming Your Anger Style Can Change Your Life.*

Healing Shame

Engel, Beverly. *It Wasn't Your Fault: Freeing Yourself from the Shame of Childhood Abuse with the Power of Self-Compassion.*
Kaufman, Gershen. *Shame: The Power of Caring.*

Domestic Violence

Bancroft, Lundy. *Should I Stay or Should I Go? A Guide to Knowing if Your Relationship Can—and Should—Be Saved.*
_____. *Why Does He Do That? Inside the Minds of Angry and Controlling Men.*

Self-Empowerment for Women

Engel, Beverly. *I'm Saying No! Standing Up Against Sexual Assault, Sexual Harassment, and Sexual Pressure.*

_____. *Loving Him Without Losing You: How to Stop Disappearing and Start Being Yourself.*

_____. *The Nice Girl Syndrome: 10 Steps to Empowering Yourself and Ending Abuse.*

Self-Compassion

Germer, C. *The Mindful Path to Self-Compassion: Freeing Yourself from Destructive Thoughts and Emotions.*

Neff, Kristin. *Self-Compassion: The Proven Power of Being Kind to Yourself.*

Borderline Personality Disorder

Kreger, Randi. *The Essential Family Guide to Borderline Personality Disorder: New Tools and Techniques to Stop Walking on Eggshells.*

Kreisman, Jerold, and Hal Straus. *I Hate You—Don't Leave Me: Understanding Borderline Personality Disorder.*

_____. *Talking to a Loved One with Borderline Personality Disorder: Communication Skills to Manage Intense Emotions, Set Boundaries, and Reduce Conflict.*

Mason, Paul T., and Randi Kreger. *Stop Walking on Eggshells: Taking Your Life Back When Someone You Care About Has Borderline Personality Disorder.*

Narcissistic Personality Disorder

Miller, Meredith. *The Journey: A Roadmap for Self-Healing After Narcissistic Abuse.*

Morningstar, Dana. *Out of the Fog: Moving from Confusion to Clarity After Narcissistic Abuse.*

Simon, J. H. *How to Kill a Narcissist: Debunking the Myth of Narcissism and Recovering from Narcissistic Abuse.*

Divorce

Eddy, Bill, and Randi Kreger. *Splitting: Protecting Yourself While Divorcing Someone with Borderline or Narcissistic Personality Disorder.*

Memoirs on Escaping Emotional or Physical Abuse

Morris, Marguerite. *Leaving: One Woman's Story of Verbal Abuse.*
Morgan Steiner, Leslie. *Crazy Love.*

Memoirs on Recovering from an Abusive and/or Neglectful Childhood

Engel, Beverly. *Raising Myself: A Memoir of Neglect, Shame, and Growing Up
    Too Soon.*
Wisechild, Louise. *The Mother I Carry: A Memoir of Healing from Emotional
    Abuse.*

References

Chapter 1: Emotional Abuse and Shame—A Perfect Marriage

Karakurt, Günnur, and Kristin Silver. 2013. "Emotional Abuse in Intimate Relationships: The Role of Gender and Age." *Violence and Victims* 28, no. 5: 804–21.

Turner, Mary. 2001. "Shame on You: Self-Blame Can Literally Make You Sick." www.webmd.com.

Chapter 2: Determining Whether You Are Being Emotionally Abused

Karakurt and Silver. "Emotional Abuse."

Mouzos, Jenny, and Toni Makkai. 2004. *Women's Experience of Male Violence: Findings from the Australian Component of the International Violence Against Women Survey (IVAWS)*. Canberra: Australian Institute of Criminology.

Chapter 3: Tools of the Trade

Engel, Beverly. 2007. *The Jekyll and Hyde Syndrome*. Hoboken, NJ: John Wiley & Sons.

Forward, Susan. 2019. *Emotional Blackmail*. New York: Harper Paperbacks.

Stevenson, Robert Louis. 2018. *The Strange Case of Dr. Jekyll and Mr. Hyde*. Orinda, CA: SeaWolf Press.

Chapter 4: How Shaming Works as a Means of Gaining Control

Turner. "Shame on You."

Van der Kolk, B. A. 1989. "The Compulsion to Repeat the Trauma: Reenactment, Revictimization, and Masochism." *Psychiatric Clinics of North America* 12, no. 2: 389–411.

Chapter 5: Taking Shame Out of the Situation

Chapple, C. L. 2003. "Examining Intergenerational Violence: Violent Role Modeling or Weak Parental Controls? *Violence and Victims* 18, no. 2: 143–62.

DePrince. A. P. 2005. "Social Cognition and Revictimization Risk." *Journal of Trauma and Dissociation* 6, no. 1: 125–41.

Engel, Beverly. 2015. *It Wasn't Your Fault: Freeing Yourself from the Shame of Childhood Abuse with the Power of Self-Compassion*. Oakland, CA: New Harbinger.

Gilbert, R., C. S. Widom, K. Browne, D. Fergusson, E. Webb, and S. Janson. 2009. "Burden and Consequences of Child Maltreatment in High-Income Countries." *Lancet* 373, no. 9657: 68–81.

Gobin, R. L., and J. J. Freud. 2014. "The Impact of Betrayal Trauma on the Tendency to Trust." *Psychological Trauma: Theory, Research, Practice, and Policy* 6, no. 5: 505–11.

Herman, Judith. 2015. *Trauma and Recovery: The Aftermath of Violence*. New York: Basic Books.

Kaufman, Gershen. 1992. *Shame: The Power of Caring*. Rochester, VT: Schenkman Books, Inc.

Mouzos and Makkai. *Women's Experience of Male Violence*.

Norman, R. E., M. Byambaa, R. De, A. Butchart, J. Scott J., and T. Vos. 2012. "The Long-Term Health Consequences of Child Physical Abuse, Emotional Abuse and Neglect: A Systematic Review and Meta-analysis." *PLOS Medicine* 9, no. 11: 1–31.

Tackett, Kathleen Kendall. 2001. *The Long Shadow: Adult Survivors of Childhood Abuse*. Oakland, CA: New Harbinger.

Widom, C. S., S. Czaja, and M. A. Dutton. 2014. "Child Abuse and Neglect and Intimate Partner Violence Victimization and Perpetration: A Prospective Investigation." *Child Abuse & Neglect* 38, no. 4: 650–63.

Chapter 6: Stop Believing the Abuser

de Becker, Gavin. 1999. *The Gift of Fear: And Other Survival Signals That Protect Us from Violence*. New York: Dell.
Gilbert, P. 2005. "Compassion and Cruelty: A Biopsychosocial Approach." In *Compassion: Conceptualizations, Research, and Use in Psychotherapy*, edited by P. Gilbert. London: Routledge.
Longe, O., F. A. Maratos, P. Gilbert, G. Evans, F. Volker, H. Rockliff, and G. Rippon. 2010. "Having a Word with Yourself: Neural Correlates of Self-Criticism and Self-Reassurance." *Neuroimage* 49, no. 2: 1849–56
Shapira, Leah B., and Myriam Mongrain. 2010. "The Benefits of Self-Compassion and Optimism Exercises for Individuals Vulnerable to Depression." *Journal of Positive Psychology* 5, no. 5: 377–89.

Chapter 7: Using Your Anger to Deprogram and Empower Yourself

Levine, Peter. 1997. *Waking the Tiger: Healing Trauma*. Berkeley, CA: North Atlantic Books.

Chapter 8: Give Yourself the Gift of Self-Compassion

Neff, Kristin. 2015. *Self Compassion: The Proven Power of Being Kind to Yourself*. New York: William Morrow.
Longe et al. "Having a Word with Yourself."

Chapter 9: Is There Hope for Your Relationship?

American Psychiatric Association. 2013. *Diagnostic and Statistical Manual of Mental Disorders: Fifth Edition: DSM-5*. Washington, DC: American Psychiatric Association Publishing.

Soper, Richard G. 2014. "Intimate Partner Violence and Co-Occurring Substance Abuse/Addiction." American Society of Addiction Medicine. www.asam.org.

Chapple. "Examining Intergenerational Violence."

de Becker. *Gift of Fear.*

Engel, Beverly. 2003. *The Emotionally Abusive Relationship: How to Stop Being Abused and How to Stop Abusing.* Hoboken, NJ: John Wiley & Sons.

Gilbert et al. "Burden and Consequences of Child Maltreatment."

Kwong, M. J., K. Bartholomew, A. J. Henderson, and S. J. Trinke. 2003. "The Intergenerational Transmission of Relationship Violence." *Journal of Family Psychology* 17, no. 3: 288–301.

Mason, Paul T., and Randi Kreger. 2020. *Stop Walking on Eggshells: Taking Your Life Back When Someone You Care About Has Borderline Personality Disorder, Third Edition.* Oakland, CA: New Harbinger.

Simpson, T. L., and W. R. Miller. 2002. "Concomitance Between Childhood Sexual Abuse and Physical Abuse and Substance Use Problems. A Review." *Clinical Psychology Review* 22, no. 1: 27–77.

Whiting, J. B., L. A. Simmons, J. R. Havens, D. B. Smith, and M. Oka. 2009. "Intergenerational Transmission of Violence: The Influence of Self-Appraisals, Mental Disorders, and Substance Abuse. *Journal of Family Violence* 24: 639–48.

Widom et al. "Child Abuse and Neglect."

Chapter 10: Confronting Your Partner

de Becker. *Gift of Fear.*

Engel, Beverly. 2001. *The Power of Apology,* Hoboken, NJ: John Wiley.

Chapter 11: Indications That You Need to End the Relationship

A Conscious Rethink. 2019. "12 Ways to Spot a Malignant Narcissist in Your Life." aconsciousrethink.com.

Mayo Clinic. Mayoclinic.org/diseases/conditions/antisocialpersonality disordermayoclinic.org/diseases-conditions/antisocial-personality-disorder/symptoms-cause/syc-20353728

Chapter 12: If You Decide to Stay

Mason and Kreger. *Stop Walking on Eggshells.*

Chapter 13: Fighting the Temptation to Go Back

Bancroft. Lundy. 2003. *Why Does He Do That? Inside the Minds of Angry and Controlling Men.* New York: Berkley Books.

Levine. *Waking the Tiger.*

Chapter 14: Forgive Yourself by Understanding Yourself

Neff, 73.

Viorst, Judith. 1998. *Necessary Losses.* New York: Simon & Schuster.

Chapter 15: Continuing to Focus on Healing Your Shame

Bach, Tara. 2004. *Radical Acceptance: Embracing Your Life with the Heart of a Buddha.* New York: Bantam.

Gilbert. "Compassion and Cruelty."

Longe et al. "Having a Word with Yourself."

Levine. *Waking the Tiger.*

Neff. *Self-Compassion,* 48.

Mellin, Laurel. 2003. *The Pathway: Follow the Road to Health and Happiness.* New York: William Morris Paperbacks.

Shapira and Mongrain. "Benefits of Self-Compassion."

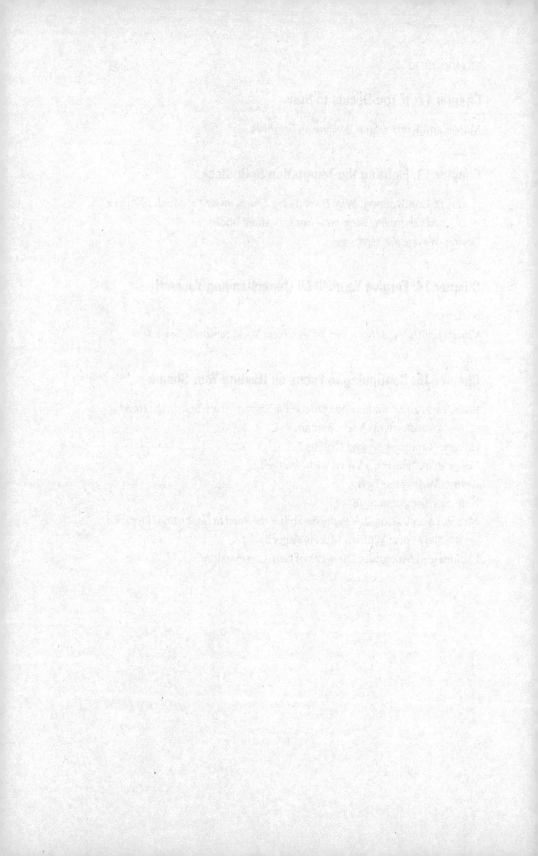

Acknowledgments

First and foremost, I want to express my gratitude to all my clients—past and present—who worked so hard to face the truth about their relationship and to heal their shame so that they could become strong enough to either confront their abuser or end the relationship. Working with you helped me to continue to fine-tune my shame reduction program so that I could help other clients, and your courage has been a constant inspiration to me.

Next, I wish to acknowledge everyone who helped in the publication process, starting with my agent, Tom Miller, and my editor, Denise Silvestro. Thank you for recognizing the importance of this book and for all your efforts to help the book come to fruition. I also want to thank Jeffrey Robert Lindholm for his copyediting as well as Barbara Brown for her cover design.

Index

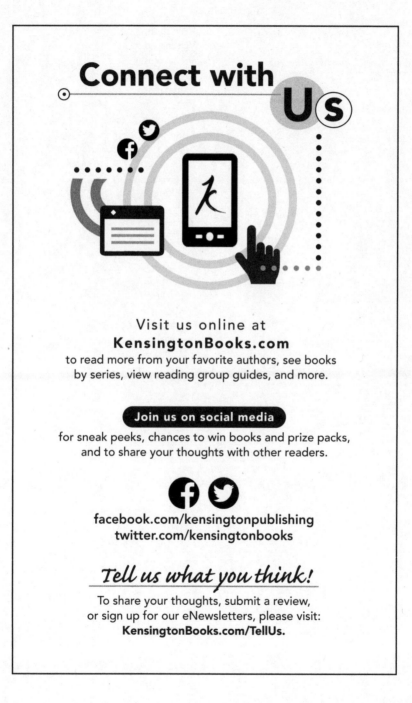

Connect with Us

Visit us online at
KensingtonBooks.com
to read more from your favorite authors, see books
by series, view reading group guides, and more.

Join us on social media

for sneak peeks, chances to win books and prize packs,
and to share your thoughts with other readers.

facebook.com/kensingtonpublishing
twitter.com/kensingtonbooks

Tell us what you think!

To share your thoughts, submit a review,
or sign up for our eNewsletters, please visit:
KensingtonBooks.com/TellUs.

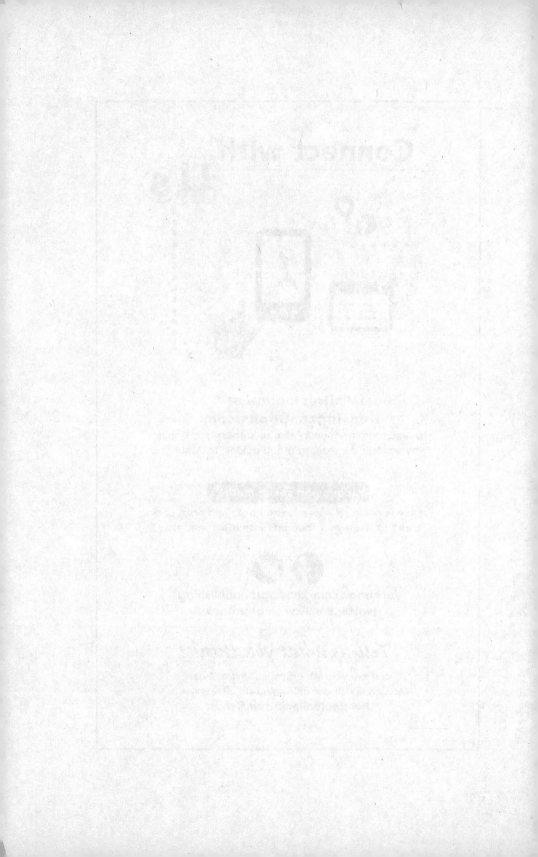